MOXA
— IN —
MOTION

WITH THE ONTAKE METHOD

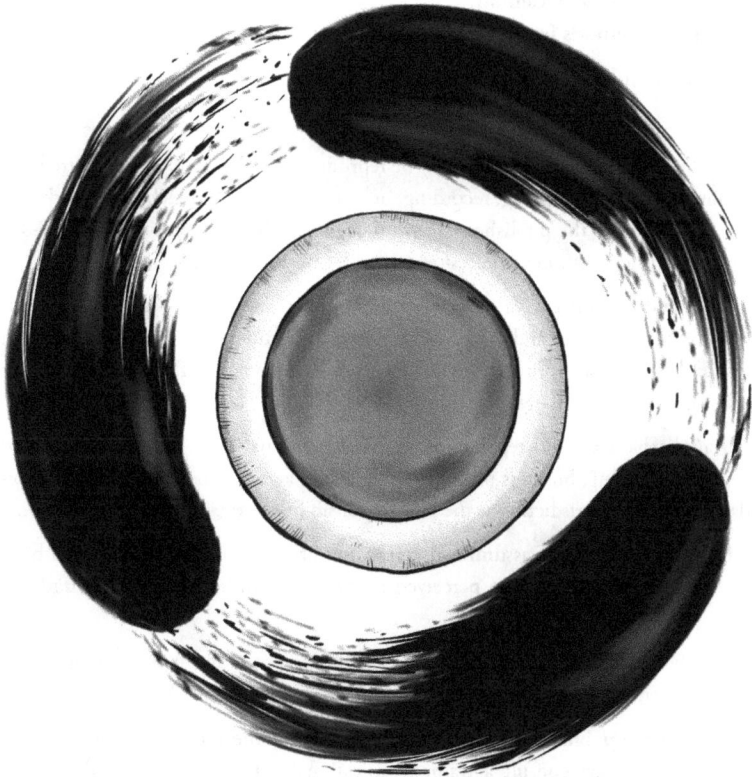

Rhythmic Moxibustion Methods from Japan
for Mind-Body Healing

ORAN KIVITY

Moxa in Motion with the Ontake Method:
Rhythmic Moxibustion Methods from Japan for Mind-Body Healing

Copyright © 2019 by Oran Kivity

Cover Design by 100Covers.com

Interior Design by FormattedBooks.com

Thank you, Billy.

You make everything possible.

Illustrations by

Vio Lau

DOWNLOAD THE COLOUR POSTER OF THE TAPPING ZONES FOR FREE!

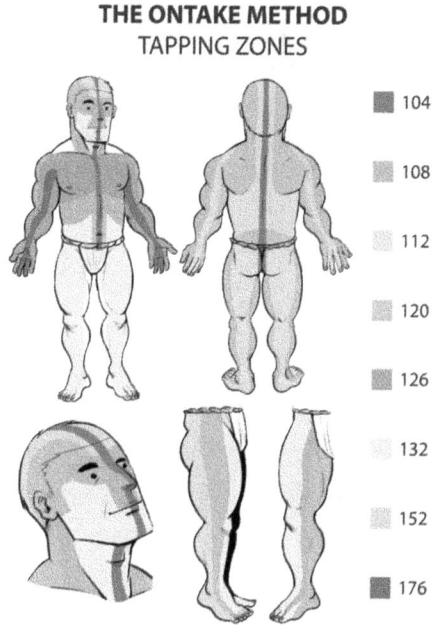

THE ONTAKE METHOD
TAPPING ZONES

104
108
112
120
126
132
152
176

© Oran Kivity 2019

THANK YOU FOR BUYING THIS BOOK.

PLEASE DOWNLOAD A COLOUR CHART OF THE TAPPING ZONES FOR FREE!

TO DOWNLOAD GO TO:
www.orankivity.com/tapme

Contents

PART 1: THE BASICS

PART 3: GOING HOLOGRAPHIC

PART 4: BAMBOO SHOOTS

CHAPTER 13: INTEGRATING ONTAKE WITH MANAKA'S FOUR-STEP PROTOCOL

CHAPTER 14: FOLLOWING MANAKA'S TRAIL

PART 1

THE BASICS

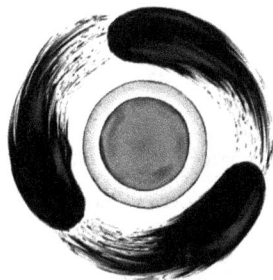

READ ME!

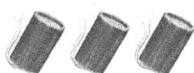

Most authors love to think that readers start their books at the beginning and read them to the end, but as an avid reader and researcher myself, I know this is not the case. If I don't read a book all the way through, then why should you?

With this in mind, I have added a chapter overview at the beginning of each chapter so that you can get a clear idea of what is there. Additionally, similar to how some restaurants add one, two, or three chilli icons to show how spicy the dishes are, each chapter starts with an Ontake rating icon to show my perspective on the content. One Ontake means "interesting", two Ontake means "very useful", and three Ontake means "essential".

Thus, there are several ways to get what you want from this book. You can:
- Skip to the practical bits
- Check the chapter headings and read what feels relevant to you
- Follow the Ontake ratings
- Read the book from cover to cover

For many reasons, I'd love you to take the fourth option and read this book from start to finish. Doing so will immerse you in Ontake and teach you a coherent approach to applying it. On the surface, this book is all about the many ways you can use Ontake to get amazing results in your clinical practice, but my ultimate intention is something more. I hope that by reading enough of the book, you become immersed in the Japanese way of approaching treatment and recognise that you can get dynamic results by being economical, what Dr Manaka described as achieving "maximum result with minimum intervention". As will be seen in the chapters on holographic systems, the body is in constant communication with itself in sometimes surprising ways. The discussions on palpation, dosage and the dynamic changes that can come about as a result of very subtle stimulation are relevant to the overall practice of acupuncture and moxibustion, even if you don't know much about Japanese acupuncture or Ontake.

Finally, Ontake changed my practice and changed my life! From the first day, I started using it, patients loved it. Ontake was not only a new clinical tool that enabled better results, but it also became a new way for me to help my patients relax. The warmth of the bamboo, the smell of the burning moxa, and the gentle ticking of the metronome all combine hypnotically to bring people into a deeply relaxed state. It is in that relaxed state that healing takes place. I suspect adopting this practice is why my patient numbers started to grow. Patients know Ontake is good for them!

Whichever way you approach this book, I hope the Ontake Method can change your practice in the same way it changed mine, leading you into a deeper understanding of palpation, moxibustion, and unspoken communication with your patients.

—Oran Kivity
Kuala Lumpur 2019

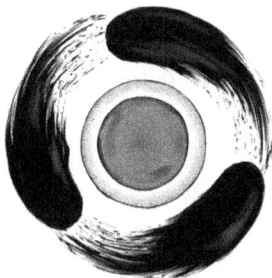

THE MAGICIAN AND THE APPRENTICE

When I begin to lecture an audience, regardless of who they are, I often begin by saying, "Don't believe what I'm going to tell you".

—*Yoshio Manaka* [1]

This book was inspired by the work of two people: the Japanese medical doctor and acupuncturist Dr Yoshio Manaka (1911–1989) and my teacher, British acupuncturist, author, and trainer Stephen Birch.

Dr Manaka was a medical doctor who combined scientific research skills with a fascination for traditional methods of healing. He was renowned in Japan during his life, working in his clinic with a team of practitioners and achieving an exceptional level of effectiveness. Always open to new concepts and ideas, he assimilated new methods into his practice—constantly researching, taking home what he found useful, and adding his own innovations and adaptations along the way. One example of this is his integration of the *Sotai* bodywork method, which uses a number of muscle stretches against resistance. Dr Manaka studied the methodology, followed it, and then added direct moxibustion to the procedure, simultaneously stretching the patient's limb with one hand and burning moxa cones with the other—a unique application of moxibustion into physical therapy.

"Don't believe what I tell you!" was Dr Manaka's catchphrase. Instead, he wanted you to believe the research. Dr Manaka placed great emphasis on researching

---

1   Manaka, Y., Itaya, K., & Birch, S. (1995). *Chasing the Dragon's Tail: The Theory and Practice of Acupuncture in the Work of Yoshio Manaka.* Brookline: Paradigm Publications, p.18.

acupuncture phenomena in experiments that could be repeated and corroborated by others. His legacy was a massive body of books and published papers in Japanese about the channel system and a coherent, methodical, and effective system of acupuncture brought to the West by Stephen Birch and Junko Ida.

Dr Manaka was fluent in ancient and modern Chinese and Japanese, French, German, and English, along with "smatterings of other languages".[2] Outside of his passion for medicine, he was a sculptor, a poet, and a painter. Thus, he was a true polymath, a medical Leonardo Da Vinci. Stephen Birch, one of the brightest lights in the Western acupuncture world, described Dr Manaka to me as the only genius he had ever met.

Dr Manaka taught Birch and corresponded with him in a process Birch described as "mind-expanding" and "exposing oneself to a kind of knowledge and curiosity virus".[3] This infection of ideas and thinking led to the English publication of *Chasing the Dragon's Tail*, written by Birch with Manaka's input and guidance. It was a seminal book on acupuncture and acupuncture research, so much so that when I came across it in a bookshop in 1989, I quickly placed it back on the shelf, thinking all those graphs and formulae were "too scientific" for me. But Birch has continued to spread the "Manaka Meme", challenging students to look at acupuncture rationally and pragmatically, testing and adapting what works, and rejecting assumptions and dogma if they don't make sense. With a doctorate in acupuncture research, Birch has been a conduit for information from Japan to the West, writing many important books about acupuncture and pushing the debate forwards about how we should study acupuncture's effects and the questions we should ask.

This book is a product of my own infection with the Manaka Meme. Without the knowledge of Manaka's meridian frequencies and the pragmatic intellectual framework for cautious experimentation and validation that Stephen Birch instilled in me, I would never have developed the Ontake Method in this form.

2   Birch, S. (2009). Dr Manaka Yoshio's Insights and Contributions to the Field of TEAM. *NAJOM Special Issue: In Memory of Dr Manaka Yoshio,* 16(47), p.18.

3   Ibid.

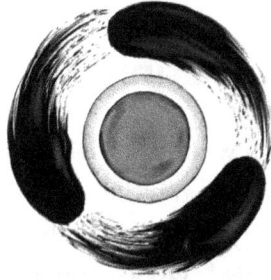

CHAPTER 1

ONTAKE ORIGINS

Introducing:

- A history of warm bamboo
- An introduction to meridian frequencies
- A personal story of inspiration and discovery

I would like to introduce another rare technique, "Bamboo Ring Moxibustion" (Takenowa Kyu 竹の輪灸). Make a long bamboo tube about 4 cm long, without a joint. The thickness of the bamboo tube wall should be about 3–4 mm. Fill it with semi-pure moxa, leaving a space at both ends of the bamboo. Compress the moxa tightly so that it can't fall out, then light it. After the bamboo gets warm, stroke the skin with it lightly and rapidly, or roll it on the affected area. ... The duration of treatment should be adjusted to the patient's condition. ... The technique can be used for supplementing and draining, just like cone moxa, so if applied correctly, it can be extremely effective for many conditions.

—Makoto Yamashita[4]

---

4 Yamashita, M. (1992). *Shinkyuchiryogaku (Acupuncture and Moxibustion Therapy)*, Tokyo, Ishiyaku Shuppan.

Definition

Meridian frequency moxibustion with Ontake is a moxibustion technique with two additional components: pressure and rhythm. A short piece of bamboo is filled with moxa wool. When the moxa is ignited, the bamboo gets hot and can be applied to the skin. The bamboo can be held, tapped, pressed, or rolled rhythmically along the acupuncture channels and on specific points. Additionally, with the use of a metronome, these techniques can be applied rhythmically at a specific number of beats per minute based on Dr Manaka's meridian frequencies. This chapter explores the origins of this treatment.

History

In 2010, I was introduced to a new moxibustion tool by Hiroshi Enomoto from Sankei acupuncture suppliers in Tokyo—a short tube of bamboo filled with moxa. It was called short bamboo and not commonly used, even in Japan. Its origins are not well documented, but it seems to be a modern development. In his recent book, moxibustion practitioner Hideo Shinma, the son of the renowned specialist of moxibustion Izaburo Fukaya, states that Zuiho Ito was the first to use it.[5] Ito was one of the students of Sorei Yanagiya, an acupuncture master in the early Showa era (1906–1959).[6] This implies that this moxibustion tool has been in use for less than a century.

In 2010, nothing had been published on bamboo ring moxibustion in English, but Mr Enomoto translated a passage for me from *Shinkyuchiryogaku (Acupuncture and Moxibustion Therapy)*, written by Makoto Yamashita in 1992.[7] Yamashita may have been using this technique as early as the 1960s.

Given how long moxibustion has existed, bamboo ring moxibustion is like a newborn baby, arriving sometime around the later part of the twentieth century. Yet, Yamashita considered it to be beneficial: "It works for pain relief and relieves inflammation. *Bamboo Ring Moxibustion* can also work for pain relief of all joint rheumatism, frozen shoulder, broken bones, and sprains. It can be applied for inflammation conditions."

---

5   Shinma H., (2012). *Take Zutsu Onkyu, (Bamboo Tube Moxibustion)*. Tokyo: Kyuho Rinsho Kenkyukai.

6   Enomoto, H. (2010, April 13). (Personal correspondence).

7   Yamashita, M. (1992). *Shinkyuchiryogaku (Acupuncture and Moxibustion Therapy)*, Tokyo: Ishiyaku Shuppan.

The treatment is extremely soothing when received. In fact, the bamboo ring moxibustion instrument quickly revolutionized my practice, fast becoming my primary approach for treating broad areas of the body and for working along the channels. Importantly, the feeling it creates delights patients, and they frequently ask for it, impressed not just by its efficacy as a clinical tool, but also by the physical comfort and relaxation it induces.

Nomenclature

Yamashita named his treatment bamboo ring moxibustion (竹の輪灸 *takenowa kyu*). In his 2012 book, Shinma Sensei called his bamboo treatment bamboo tube moxibustion (竹筒灸 *take zutsu kyu*). In the early years of selling the tool, Sankei marketed this product with yet another name, short bamboo moxibustion (短竹灸 *tan take kyu*). This is because Sankei was already selling a longer bamboo moxibustion tool known as the moxa heat reduction tool (灸熱緩和器 *kyu netsu kanwa ki*), better known in the West as Fukaya bamboo. This relatively long bamboo tube is used to reduce the pain from the heat of direct moxibustion by pressing on the surrounding skin as the moxa cone burns down. As the Fukaya bamboo was long and the newcomer was short, to distinguish one from the other, they called it short bamboo (短竹 *tan take*).

"Short bamboo" is not a very enticing name, however—certainly not evocative at all of the warmth and relaxation induced by the therapy. So, with the help of a Japanese patient, in my own practice, I rebranded it as warm bamboo (温竹 *ontake*). *On* is the same character found in 温泉 *onsen,* "hot spring". As I started to write about *Ontake,* the new name stuck, and now Sankei enthusiastically promotes its Ontake range.

When writing about techniques developed by Yamashita Sensei or Shinma Sensei, I will refer to them as bamboo ring or bamboo tube moxibustion. In most contexts, however—particularly those concerned with meridian frequency moxibustion—I will refer to Ontake, or more simply, bamboo.

Cycles and Frequencies

Long ago, in an era far, far away, I lay on a treatment table in front of a class during the second part of my training in Manaka Style Acupuncture (MSA) with Junko Ida. Junko was demonstrating *okyu* (small cone moxibustion), and I was the model. With a speed and fluidity that I still cannot match, she applied small cones of moxa on one point on my leg. I could feel pulses of warmth that came and went, surging and receding at regular intervals. It felt fantastic, and it was at this moment that I realized the application of heat is only one component of effective moxibustion, the other being cyclical rhythm. I learnt a wordless lesson that day and rooted in the memory of my muscles, one that I never forgot.

In fact, no matter the method of application, moxibustion is by nature both cyclical and rhythmic. When burning small cones, there is a short cycle between lighting the cone, the moment when the heat peaks, and the moment when you extinguish the cone and start over. With larger cones, the cycle is longer, but when the heat peaks, the cone is still removed and replaced. With warm needle technique, the cones are burnt on the needle, and the cycle is even slower. With this kind of technique, the frequency is lower.

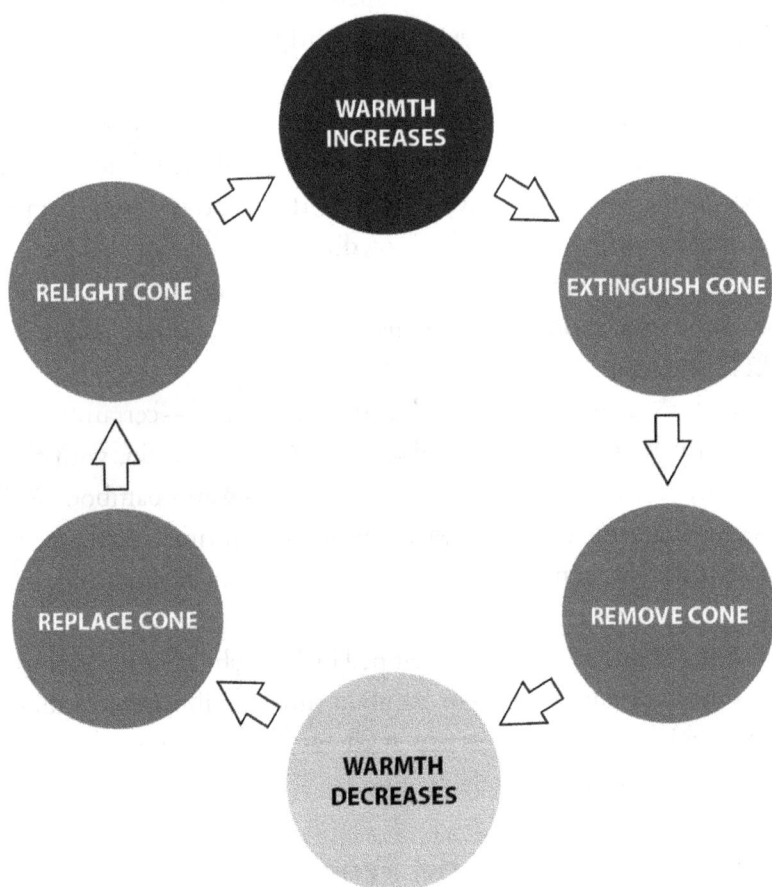

All moxibustion is cyclical.

On the other end of the spectrum, in Chinese therapy, moxa sticks are applied with a relatively high-frequency, rhythmic, sparrow-pecking motion. Warmth is applied and removed rhythmically. Given that we are dealing with the application of heat, it makes total sense to remove the heat periodically. The skin cannot take a heat source indefinitely without pain or injury. It needs periods of rest, so the heat must be applied and removed. These cycles can be short or long, depending on the nature of the heat source.

Dr Manaka and Meridian Frequencies

The application of treatment with rhythm and frequency has a long pedigree in Traditional East Asian Medicine (TEAM), both in bodywork and acupuncture. In my early years of practice, I studied Tui Na, where the primary stroke is rolling: a supple, rhythmic oscillation of the wrist. In Zen Shiatsu, there is a stroke called Vibrating, where the hand oscillates very rapidly while placed on the area to be treated.

In sixteenth century Japan, a physician named Isai Misono developed the percussive acupuncture style of the Mubunryu school. This practice involved lightly tapping thick needles with a wooden mallet on reactive points on the abdomen.[8] The Japanese word *shin* is translated as "needle" in English, but in these tapping styles, the needle was in fact a blunt gold or silver probe. Following this tradition, twentieth century Japanese doctor and acupuncturist Yoshio Manaka developed percussive tapping treatments using his own wooden hammer and needle designs.[9] Using a needle made of wood instead of gold and not restricting himself to points on the abdomen, Manaka tapped lightly on the acupuncture channels to stimulate the flow of qi, relieving muscle tightness and easing pain. He developed this technique to treat a wide range of symptoms and also taught patients to perform it at home as a self-administered therapy.

He focused this work further by researching specific frequencies (in beats per minute) for each acupuncture channel. When tapping channels at various frequencies, he noted beneficial effects on pressure pain at the diagnostic front-*mu* points on the abdomen. In other words, by tapping on a point on the arm or leg at a specific frequency, he could make a diagnostic point on the abdomen softer. Tapping with other frequencies would not get the same effect.

---

8   Birch, S., & Ida, J. (1998). *Japanese Acupuncture, A Clinical Guide.* Brookline: Paradigm Publications, p. 4.

9   Manaka, Y., Itaya, K., & Birch, S. (1995). *Chasing the Dragon's Tail: The Theory and Practice of Acupuncture in the Work of Yoshio Manaka.* Brookline: Paradigm Publications.

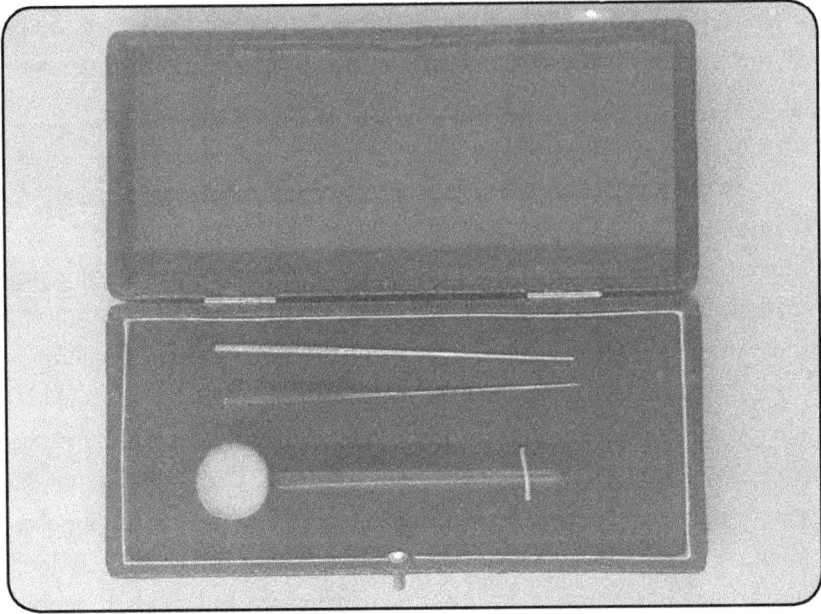

Mubunryu gold needle and hammer.[10]

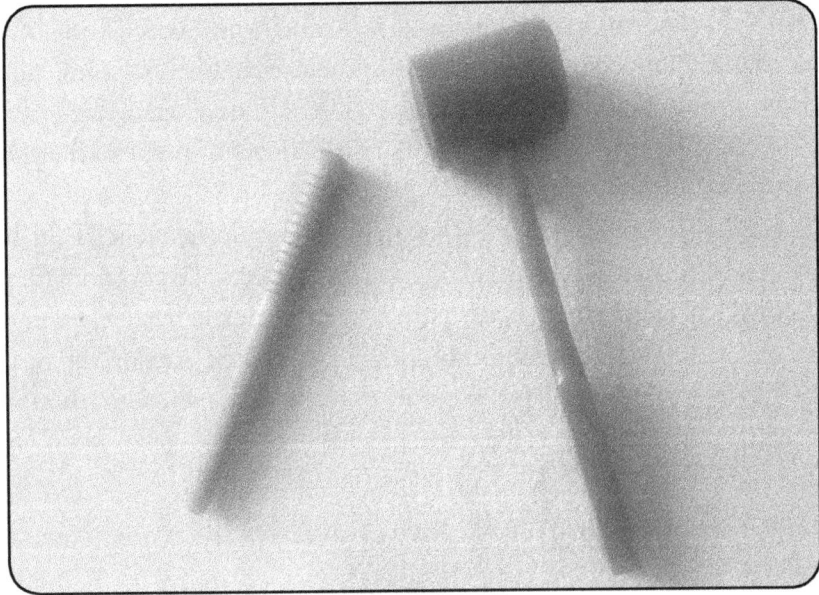

Manaka wooden needle and hammer.

In Japanese acupuncture, releasing tight points on the abdomen is regarded as a therapeutic Holy Grail, and by researching the effects of tapping in this way, Manaka

---

10   Photo courtesy the Harikyu Museum (Museum of Traditional Medicine) Osaka, Japan.

was able to chart frequencies for all twelve main acupuncture channels and two of the Eight Extraordinary Vessels, the Governor and Conception vessels.

This advanced the efficacy and range of application of his wooden hammer and needle considerably, and it became an important part of his well-known four-step protocol of treatment, later disseminated to the West by Stephen Birch and Junko Ida.

Ontake and Meridian Frequencies

I had already been fascinated by the efficacy of the wooden hammer and Manaka's meridian frequencies as treatment tools, particularly when applied to open points (*zi wu liu zhu* and *ling gui ba fa*). Always mindful that the application of heat must be rhythmic, I experimented with a moxa stick, sparrow pecking at Dr Manaka's meridian frequencies. However, I found problems with this method. The heat produced by a moxa stick is radiant and therefore there is no direct contact with the skin, losing an essential component of Manaka's original percussive method.

There are methods of applying moxa sticks with direct contact, however, and I became adept at press moxibustion *shi'an jiu* or its Japanese equivalent *oshi kyu*. These methods involve pressing the hot tip along the channels, with a few layers of newspaper or cloth to insulate the patients from burns.[11] Junji Mizutani, a moxibustion specialist based in Canada, described a case where he pressed a moxa stick on all the yang channels of a cold and yang-deficient patient, achieving excellent results.[12] Press moxibustion is a dynamic and effective treatment method, but it is fraught with difficulties, not least of which are setting fire to the insulating material or dropping red hot ash on the floor.

Unlike a moxa stick, Ontake can be pressed directly on the skin. It can be rolled, tapped, and knocked with considerable force without dislodging any ash. While there is still no direct contact between the burning moxa and the skin, there is heat conduction, indirect radiation, and a range of effects on the soft tissue from the physical contact of the bamboo, such as compression and stretching.

If you hold a piece of bamboo flat in your hand, it naturally rocks forwards and back. A cylinder is inherently rhythmic. Thus, both the cylindrical shape of bamboo and its application as a moxibustion tool suggest rhythm. A rhythm requires a frequency that is either high or low, fast or slow. When introduced to Ontake, it was love at first sight. Bamboo was the tool I had been looking for. I was immediately

---

11   Auteroche, B. (1992). *Acupuncture and Moxibustion: A Guide to Clinical Practice*. Edinburgh: Churchill Livingstone.

12   Mizutani, J. (1998). Practical Moxibustion Therapy. *North American Journal of Oriental Medicine*. Canada.

inspired to combine the rhythmic strokes suggested by its size and shape with Dr Manaka's meridian frequencies.

With Tui Na as an early influence in my TEAM education, I developed a series of light and supple strokes with which to apply bamboo. When these were applied at Dr Manaka's meridian frequencies, I was amazed at the results. When heat is applied to the channels at their respective frequencies, it extends the range of therapeutic effects offered by the wooden hammer and needle. The changes in soft tissue tension are very rapid and feel deeply relaxing to patients. This led to the development of a rapidly expanding repertoire of branch treatments, as well as a whole-body root treatment. More recently, I integrated new ways of applying Ontake for pain relief using various holographic acupuncture models, including Manaka's octahedral model of the body, and adaptations of Dr Tan's Balance Method and Hirata's zones. These methods have produced wonderful results for the rapid relief of pain and will be discussed in full later.

Since the original bamboo moxibustion technique was called bamboo ring moxibustion, it seemed appropriate to call this frequency-enhanced method meridian frequency moxibustion. Meridian frequency moxibustion with Ontake has hugely expanded the range of possibilities for bamboo treatment and has been the focus of much of my writing and teaching in the last few years. The following chapters examine its many uses in the clinic.

Summary

Within the long tradition of acupuncture, bamboo is the new kid on the block. It is a historical newcomer and a brand-new addition to the acupuncturist's toolkit. It is used as a pressing and rolling tool that also delivers both radiant and conducted heat. The addition of Manaka's meridian frequencies broadens its range and scope. In the next chapter, we explore the practical aspects of how to get started.

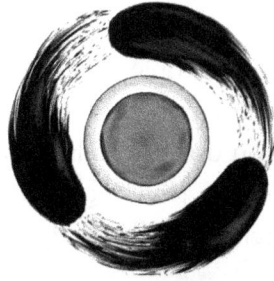

CHAPTER 2

GETTING STARTED

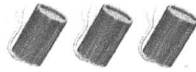

Covering all the practical aspects of sourcing, loading, and lighting bamboo.

Make a long bamboo tube about 4 cm long, without a joint. The thickness of the bamboo tube wall should be about 3–4 mm. Fill it with semi-pure moxa, leaving a space at both ends of the bamboo.

—Makoto Yamashita[13]

Ontake is like a traditional moxa box, but much smaller and more mobile. It is versatile and effective, especially when applied with Dr Manaka's meridian frequencies. You can be agile and flexible, treating small or broad areas quickly, and patients find the experience comfortable and soothing. What's more, performing Ontake is simple. Even without any theory or training, tapping or rolling a piece of warm bamboo on someone's tight shoulders can get good results.

My aim in writing this book is to make Ontake as practical as possible. While the length of this book makes clear that there is much theory to discuss and share, I know

---

13   Yamashita, M. (1992). *Shinkyuchiryogaku (Acupuncture and Moxibustion Therapy)*. Tokyo: Ishiyaku Shuppan.

from teaching workshops that some people prefer to simply pick up the bamboo and get started. For this reason, I want to start the book with practicalities and move into theory and applications later. You don't need knowledge of holographic models to get started. You don't even need a metronome to get started. You just need a single Ontake, some moxa, and a lighter. You will learn quickly that Ontake feels warm and relaxing, wherever you apply it.

Making Your Bamboo

Bamboo is easy to obtain. Nearly any garden centre can sell you a long length that you can cut into many pieces of varying sizes. You'll need a fine-toothed saw that can cut into the smooth surface of the bamboo without splintering it and a metal file or rasp. Use the file to create a tapered, blunt lip on each end of the tube. It is very important to get rid of any sharp edges on the lip of the bamboo, because you will use the blunted edge to press down on the meridians or points.

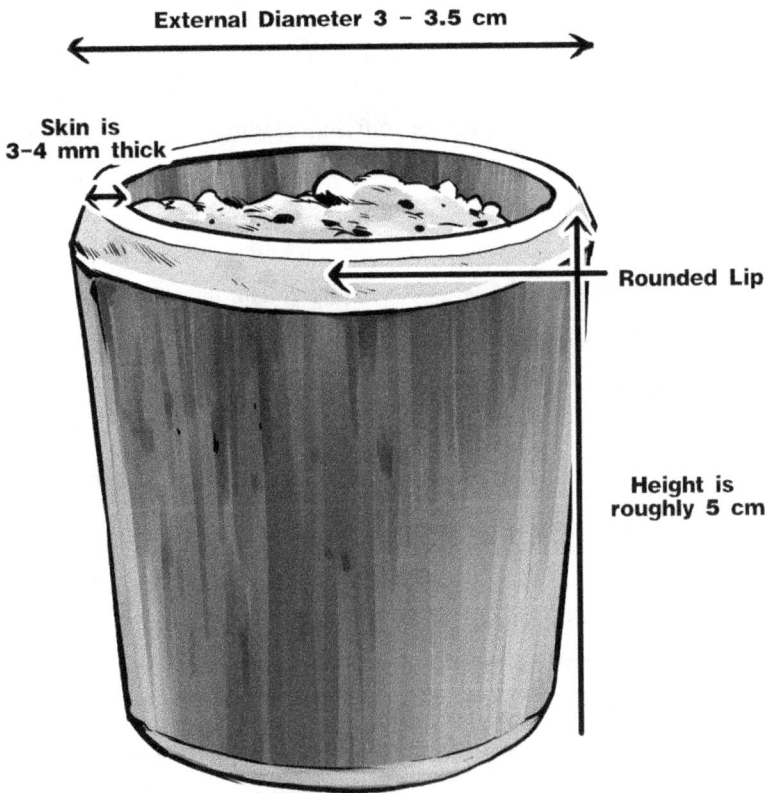

External Diameter 3 – 3.5 cm

Skin is 3–4 mm thick

Rounded Lip

Height is roughly 5 cm

Ontake dimensions.

The handmade Ontake supplied by Sankei acupuncture suppliers in Tokyo are about 5 centimetres long and 3 to 3.5 centimetres across—slightly larger than Yamashita's description above. This means you should choose your bamboo pole from the garden centre carefully. It shouldn't be too narrow or too thick. Of course, bamboo poles grow thick at the base and taper at the top, so you may have to "top and tail" it, cutting away the narrow top and the thickened base to get to the right dimensions in the middle. The narrowest useable part can be used to make mini-Ontake (see below).

The length of the tube in relation to the diameter of the bore is quite important. If the bore is too narrow, or if the length is too long, the moxa will be hard to pack and won't breathe when burning, meaning that you will have to relight it continually during treatment. If the bore is too wide, then you'll have to pack in much more moxa for a tight fit. In that case, the bamboo becomes an expensive vehicle, like a fuel-inefficient car, and it may get overly hot.

The final factor to consider is the thickness of the skin. If it's very thick, the bamboo won't get warm enough to do its magic. If it's too thin, the bamboo will become uncomfortably hot, so you'll need to cover the treatment area with a thin cloth and change your grip frequently to minimise your own discomfort.

The more you use a piece of bamboo, the thinner the skin will get, charring gradually over weeks and months from the inside out. Eventually, it will start getting too hot, get hot too quickly, or develop longitudinal cracks. Once any of those happen, you'll reluctantly have to put it into retirement.

It is worth mentioning that Felip Caudet, a physiotherapist and moxibustion practitioner in Spain, has developed the Superontake, a longer bamboo tube that can be five to eight centimetres in length. The extra length gives more leverage when pressing and is also cool to hold at one end.

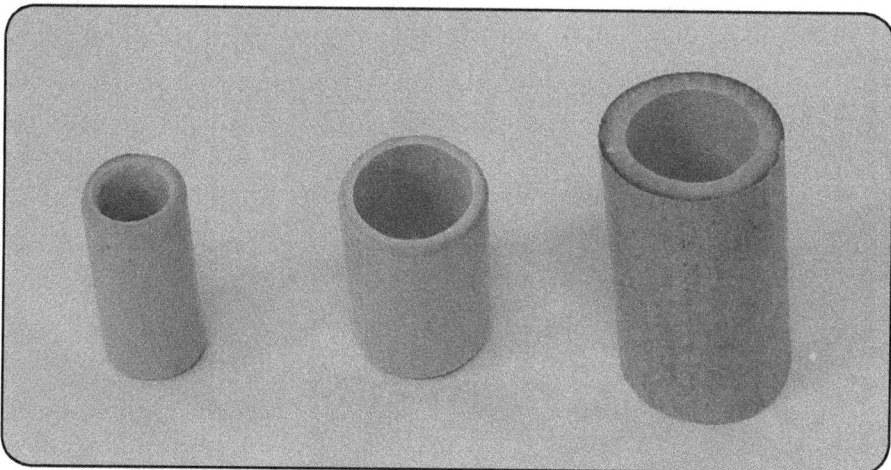

From left to right: mini-Ontake, Ontake, Superontake.

I also keep a selection of smaller bamboo called mini-Ontake that are narrower in bore than the standard variety described above. These are very useful for treating children and for treating the face, especially when going near the eyes. Some patients, understandably, get nervous when you bring heated, smouldering tools near their eyes. Mini-Ontake are less hot and much less threatening than standard sizes. However, since the bore is narrower, they breathe less easily and need to be relit frequently.

Bamboo Anatomy

Different techniques described in this book refer to different parts of the bamboo, so it is useful to define each part.

Table 1. Bamboo Anatomy

Part	Description
Mouth	The circular openings at each end of the bamboo. Caudet calls the lighted mouth the primary mouth and the unlit mouth the secondary mouth.
Shaft/Side	The side of the bamboo, the part that you roll with.
Skin	The thickness of the shaft. The skin is charred and rough on the inside and smooth on the outside. With constant use, the bamboo's skin gets thinner and thinner.
Lip	The blunted edge of the mouth. Important for focused pressing.
Bore	The circular inner tube of the bamboo. The wider the bore, the more moxa your bamboo will use. The narrower the bore, the less air will get to the plug.
Plug	The compressed moxa in the bore. The moxa should not be too tightly compressed, or the plug will not be able to breathe. Conversely, it should not be too loose, or the plug may fall out.
Base	The mouth of the bamboo facing downwards. Another term for the primary mouth.

Buying Bamboo

There is definitely some satisfaction in making and using your own bamboo, but if you're not confident about making your own, then you can order Ontake online.*[14] I actually prefer Sankei's handcrafted bamboo to my own homemade versions, perhaps because the kind of bamboo I can source here in Malaysia does not look or feel as good as the bamboo from Japan. Sankei's Ontake are not expensive, considering how much time it takes to make a good job of sanding the ends down. Mr Enomoto makes normal Ontake, and Superontake are handmade by Shinma Sensei himself.

Types of Moxa

In many Ontake techniques, the bamboo is held vertically on the skin, so we need to use a semi-pure moxa that does not drop heated particles onto the patient. Wakakusa semi-pure moxa, made by Yamasho and commonly sold in the West for large cone moxa and *kyutoshin* (warm needle), is suitable for this purpose. In fact, it is too good. If you have it, you can certainly use it with total confidence, but I have happily used Myojo moxa, also by Yamasho, which is slightly less pure, much cheaper, but just as safe. In my experience, anything less pure than Myojo is too coarse. I avoid green Chinese moxa wools, which are very twiggy and dusty.

What's great about Ontake is that it can be used to recycle partly used moxa cones from your *chinetsukyu* (cone moxa) treatments. When burning *chinetsukyu*, we typically burn down the top third or half of the cone, and when the patient feels heat, we discard the rest into a bowl of water to extinguish it. That means if we buy a 300-gram box of Wakakusa moxa, we actually throw away 150 to 200 grams. These discarded half-cones can now be collected, dried, and recycled into the ever-hungry mouth of your Ontake. Start loading the bamboo with used and dried cones, then pack both ends with new moxa to keep everything in place. This is a dirty task, so wear gloves or be prepared to clean black ash from under your nails afterwards.

Method and Techniques

Getting Started

1. Loosely fill the whole bamboo until both ends are overflowing with moxa.
2. Compress the moxa at both ends with your fingers or a small piece of wood doweling, packing roughly to the middle three-quarters of the bamboo. The

---

*14   For a list of resources, see appendix.

edge of the moxa plug should not be flush with either end of the bamboo. If packed right to the edge, it will get too hot. Too far from the edge, and it will be too cool. I have found the most effective distance to be 0.3 to 0.7cm from each end.

It is important to compress the moxa in the bamboo to stop loose moxa from falling out during treatment, or even worse, the whole plug dropping onto the skin. The bore on a new Ontake should be very smooth, and for your initial burn, you need to pack the plug relatively tightly. However, once you've used the Ontake a few times, the inner wall of the bore will have expanded and become rough. This is great for keeping the moxa in place, so you will not need to pack it quite as much.

3. You can do a simple safety test by holding the bamboo horizontally between the thumb and third finger of both hands and then inserting your index fingers into both openings. If you push the plug of moxa to the left with one finger and then to the right with the other, you can test its stability. With moderate pressure, it should not move in either direction.

Conversely, it's good not to overpack the moxa too tightly, or the plug won't breathe during combustion.

4. Light the moxa. The best way to light it is with a jet lighter, such as those used for scorching crème brûlée. The advantage of using a jet lighter is that you can get the moxa inside the bamboo to ignite very quickly. A disadvantage is that it can also overheat the lip of the bamboo to an uncomfortable temperature. Once the moxa is glowing, you need to do a second safety check before you start treatment.

Touch the bamboo on your skin in two places: first, on the palm of your hand, which is relatively insensitive. If that is OK, and if you are sure it is not too hot, try the side of your neck. The skin on your neck is relatively sensitive, so if the bamboo is tolerable on your own neck, you will not burn or startle your patient when you start treatment. Only if you are confident that the bamboo is not too hot should you apply it to the appropriate channels.

Children have much more sensitive skin than leathery, old acupuncturists, so even if it feels OK on your neck, it may not feel OK on a child. When treating children, you must start with even more caution.

5. Apply rhythmic strokes, either silently or using a metronome, according to the channel frequencies of the treatment area. Keep blowing on the bamboo to keep it burning, or relight it if it goes out.

6. To extinguish, stand the lit base of the bamboo on a level, heat-resistant surface and cover the top to cut off its oxygen. I had several methods of extin-

guishing bamboo, but last year I finally hit on the simplest. Just place a cupping jar over the bamboo, and it will run out of oxygen in a very short time.

7. For the next session, relight the bamboo from the same end. Before you relight it, put a finger in each end to check how much unburned moxa remains in the bamboo. You can judge the thickness and quality of the remaining moxa very easily this way. This procedure is only suitable for bamboo that has been extinguished for a while. Please don't poke your finger into hot ash! I often refill the bamboo at this point, without removing the unburned moxa. I simply "top up".

My colleague Marian Fixler developed her own variation of topping up, which I call the dental method. When the bamboo has cooled, she uses a probe or a plastic acupuncture guide tube to scrape out the burnt ash, a bit like a dentist drilling a tooth to get rid of decay. She then tops up the cavity with a healthy filling of fresh moxa. In my clinic, I have a dedicated tool for this—an old ice cream stick—but any long, thin object will do.

At a certain point, usually at the beginning of the week, I remove all the moxa from the bamboo and start afresh with new moxa. Frequent loading and compression start to affect the way the plug breathes. To remove the entire plug, simply hold the bamboo over a receptacle and push a small piece of wooden doweling into the top end. The plug will slowly emerge from the other end. Use the dowel to scrape the sides until the bore is completely clear, then reload.

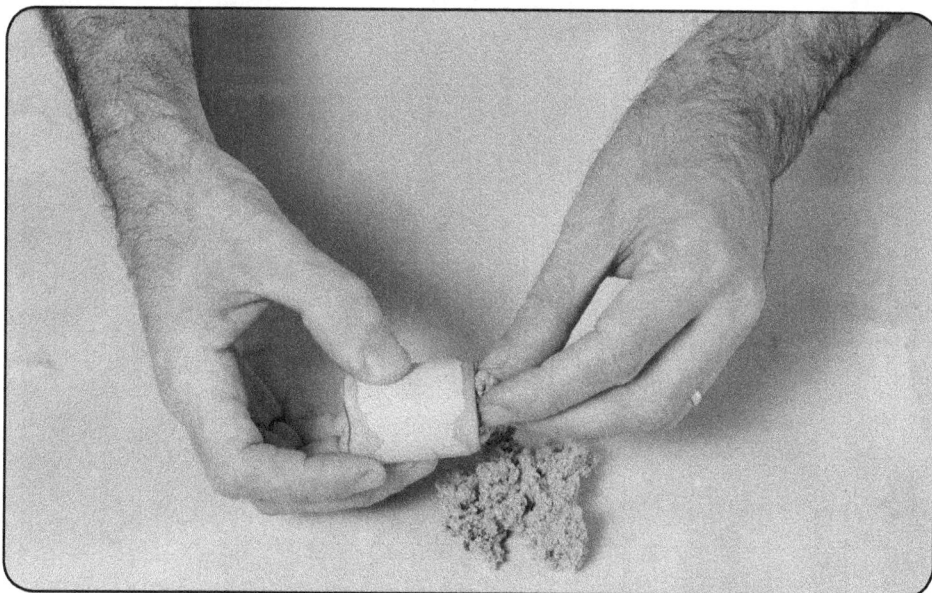

Loosely fill the Ontake until it is brimming with moxa.

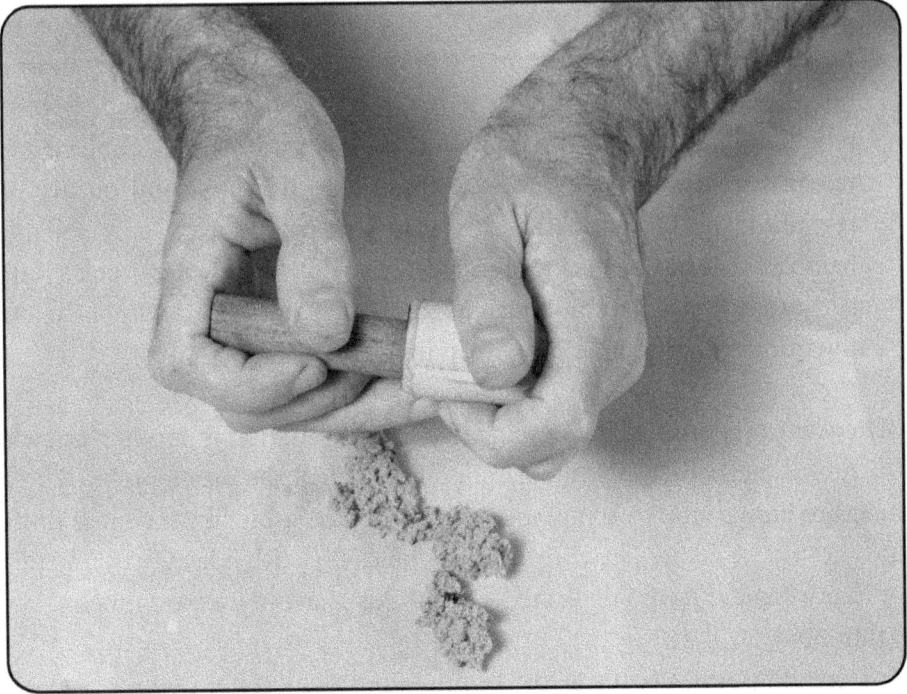

Compress the moxa with your fingers or a wooden dowel.

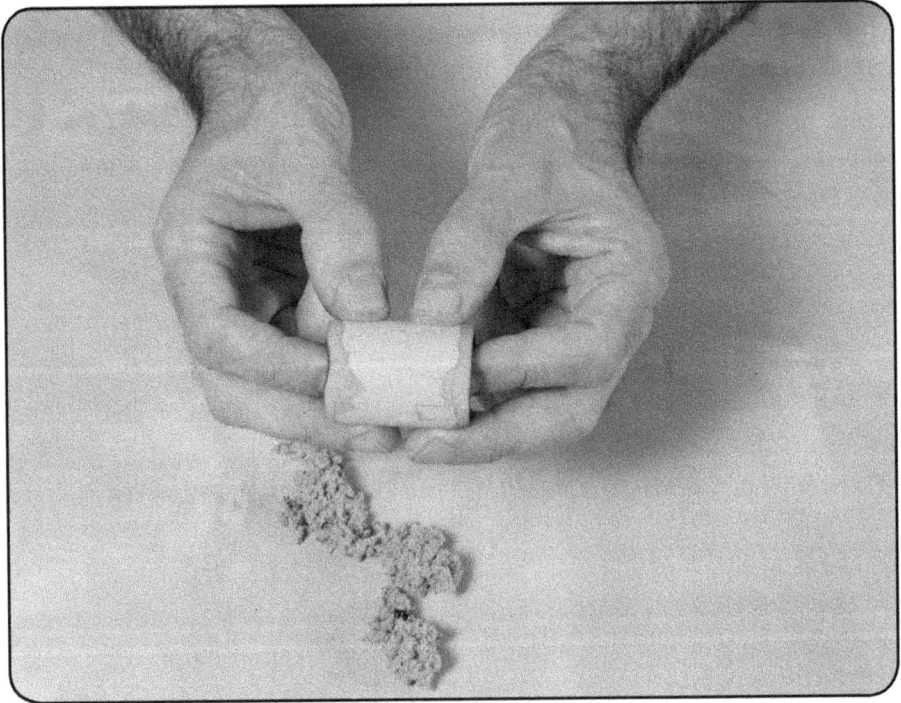

Safety test. The plug should not move easily.

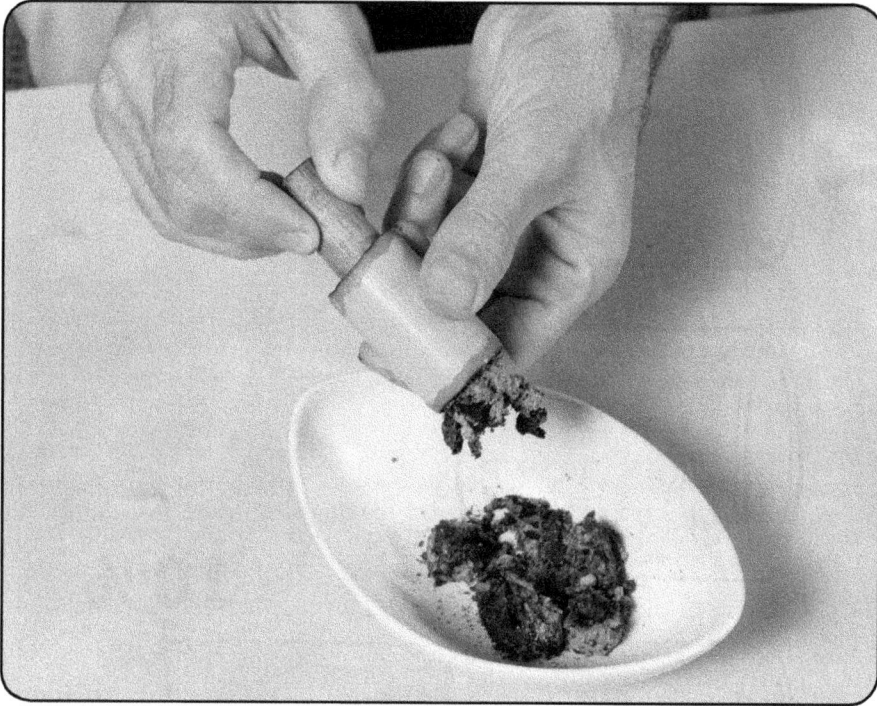

Expelling the plug with the dowel.

Yamashita, Shinma, and Caudet

It is worth mentioning that the directions above are my own take on loading bamboo. Yamashita and Shinma are both more conservative with the amount of moxa they put into the bamboo, compressing it tightly into a plug in the centre of the shaft, with a much longer gap from the lip to the burning edge of the plug. This warms the bamboo without getting it hot. For my part, I prefer the bamboo to feel quite hot at the lighted end, controlling the amount of heat the patient perceives by moderating the strokes and length of skin contact. However, some practitioners find this method makes the bamboo too hot to hold comfortably, in which case it makes more sense to use less moxa.

Felip Caudet's longer Superontake is customised to be the width of the practitioner's hand; thus, it is approximately twice the length of a normal Ontake. This length, 5 to 8 centimetres, gives extra leverage for use as a bodywork tool. The extra length also necessitates different procedures for loading, so the moxa plug is placed at one end only, and only 40% of the bamboo is filled to avoid overheating the bamboo. For practitioners with sensitive hands, this modification is great, because one end always stays cool.

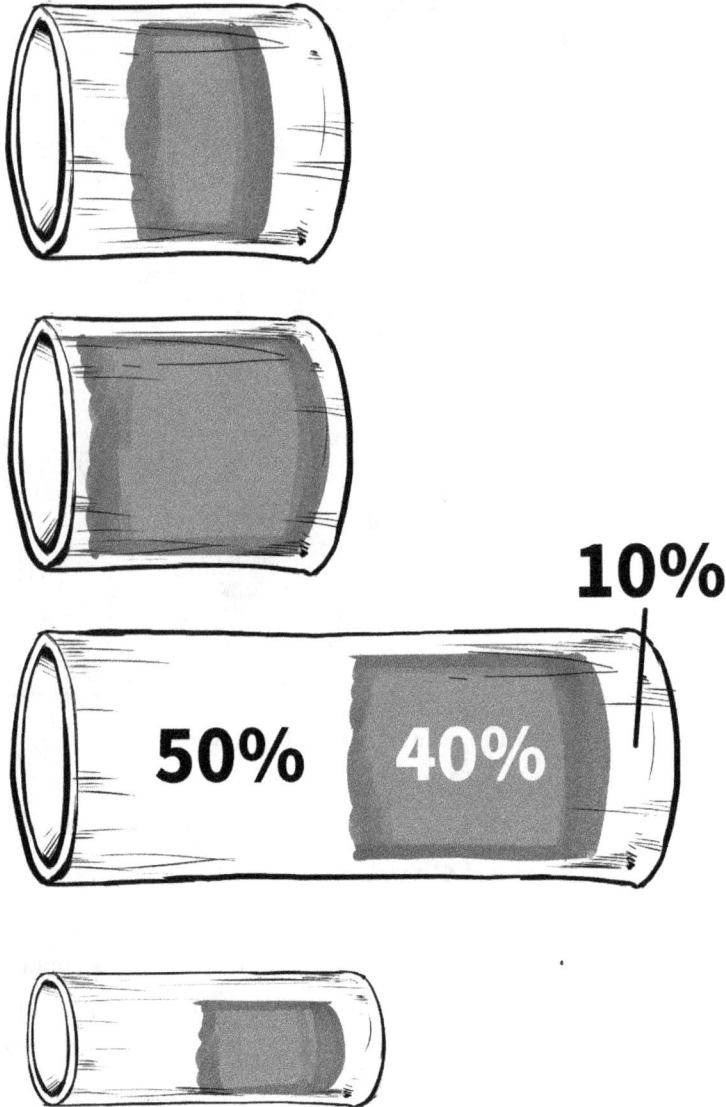

From top to bottom: Ontake loaded with central plug (Shinma and Yamashita); plug size variation (Kivity); Superontake (Caudet); mini-Ontake (Kivity).

Smoke-Free Alternatives

Surprisingly, Ontake does not generate much smoke and can be used comfortably in rooms with closed doors and windows. The only time it does get smoky is when the plug burns all the way through from one end to the other. If you allow this to happen, the amount of smoke released increases considerably and becomes noticeably more acrid.

My former assistant Koki Takemoto now works in a clinic in New Zealand equipped with smoke alarms, so Ontake is not an option. He has experimented with applying hot stones heated in water (the same as for hot stones therapy). At first, he was quite enthusiastic, but later he reported that this variation simply did not affect the body as well as bamboo. Something about the living quality of burning moxa has a more significant therapeutic effect than merely massaging the channels with warm stones, even with Manaka's dynamic meridian frequencies. This is an interesting observation, because it tells us that there may be something about the radiant heat signature of burning moxa that is therapeutic in itself.

Clinic Hygiene

It used to be applied following shiraku *treatment.*

—Hideo Shinma[15]

Moxibustion following *shiraku* (bloodletting) is still common practice in Japan. For example, this practice is taught in Toyohari as a way to stop post-treatment leaking of blood. Large cones are burnt over the site where bloodletting was performed, usually retained until the first third has burnt away. After this, the cones should be removed, placed on a metal surface, and allowed to burn down completely. However, using Ontake on the skin after *shiraku* in the same way cannot be considered a safe procedure. Certainly, if the bamboo comes into contact with blood, it should not be used again, as the porous bamboo wood cannot be effectively sterilised. It would be better to throw it away and start using a new one.

However, this does raise the issue of how to clean the bamboo. It does not break the skin and is only applied lightly on the surface, so in theory, it no more poses a health risk than your general practitioner's stethoscope touching your skin. But what if you use bamboo on someone's feet? Is it OK to use it on the next person's face without cleaning it? What constitutes effective cleaning?

The acupuncture governing bodies in different countries will answer these questions differently. In the UK, the British Acupuncture Council (BAcC) tends to regulate things quite stringently. Eventually, if Ontake becomes more common, local regulating bodies will inevitably want to legislate.

I think it's wise to consider bamboo hygiene, but we should not get too caught up with worrying about infection risks. No common bacteria could live inside the

---

15   Shinma, H. (2012). *Take Zutsu Onkyu, (Bamboo Tube Moxibustion)*. Tokyo: Kyuho Rinsho Kenkyuka. p.8

bamboo when the moxa is lit, so our only concern should be with the lip and the skin. The sides and lip of a well-made bamboo should be smooth and rounded. The technique involves making light contact with the skin, with no scratching, piercing, or rubbing until the skin is red, as in *gua sha*. Bamboo should not be used over broken skin.

Certainly, I think it's important to have a collection of preloaded bamboo to use on different people throughout the day and to wipe down the outer part of the bamboo regularly with a baby wipe. In some cases, I have soaked the bamboo in Milton Sterilising Fluid (used for babies' equipment), but soaking bamboo in liquid and then burning hot stuff inside it tends to create cracks and shorten the bamboo's lifespan.

One final option suggested by a practitioner in Germany is to use a UV sterilising cabinet, such as those used by barbers and manicurists for their tools. This can be used to sterilise and store bamboo so that a clean set is ready at the start of each day. I have started to use a UV cabinet myself. At the end of the day, I put my entire collection of used bamboo in there and let the timer bathe them in UV light for thirty minutes.*[16]

Summary

You can buy bamboo online or make your own. It can come in various lengths and sizes to accommodate different patients and practitioners. There are also best practices for loading, lighting, extinguishing, topping up, and relighting moxa in bamboo.

Bamboo feels great to receive, and it's so instinctive to use that there is nothing to stop you from starting with it right away. But what is the purpose of Ontake treatment? How does it ease pain? The next chapter explores some considerations to focus your application.

---

*16   For a list of resources, see appendix.

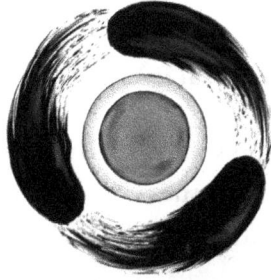

CHAPTER 3

REGULATION

Introducing Manaka's octahedral model and reviewing several concepts in the context of bamboo: yin and yang; qi and blood; deficiency and excess; supplementing and draining; and root and branch.

Defining the fundamental purpose of Ontake—the regulation of qi and blood.

The goal of meridian-based hari *therapy* (acupuncture) *is the regulation of* ki *and* ketsu *[qi and blood]. Therefore, in this form of medicine, illness is seen as disturbances in the ki and ketsu, while health is recognized as their balance.*

—*Kodo Fukushima*[17]

17   Fukushima, K. (1991). *Meridian Therapy.* Tokyo: Toyo Hari Medical Association, p.37.

Yin-Yang

The concepts of yin and yang are so ubiquitous they've almost become cliché. The purpose of this chapter is to revisit these fundamentals and other key concepts in Japanese acupuncture in the context of Ontake.

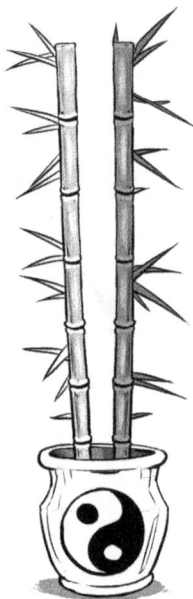

The yin-yang symbol represents two interdependent, equal, and opposite forces.

The yin-yang symbol represents two interdependent, equal, and opposite forces that are in perpetual dynamic equilibrium. In the natural world, these can be taken to mean shifting states (such as night and day, winter and summer, cold and heat and stillness and movement) or directions (such as down and up, earth and heaven, backwards and forwards). Yin-yang theory is so all-encompassing that any phenomenon in nature or the cosmos can be discussed in its terms, from the growth of a humble mould on cheese to the expanding and contracting life cycle of a sun.

Dr Manaka's Octahedral Model

Dr Manaka had pragmatic, structural interpretations of yin-yang theory. He used it to contextualise the axes of the body. The body has three axes: a vertical one that divides left from right, another vertical line that divides front and back, and a horizontal line that divides top from bottom. In anatomy, these are commonly referred to as the sagittal, coronal and transverse planes.

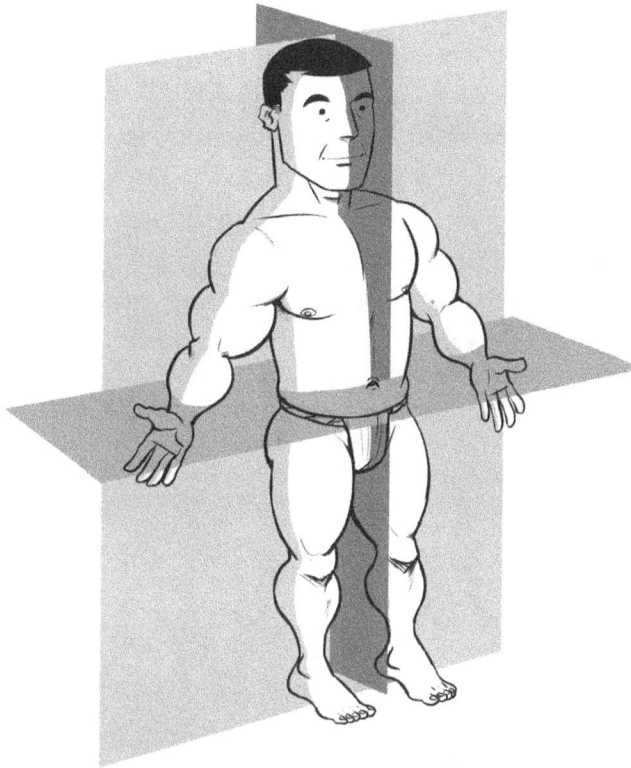

The three axes of the body create four anterior quadrants and
four posterior quadrants: an octahedral structure.

Manaka observed that if you join the ends of the three axes together, you get an octahedron, a shape described by Buckminster Fuller as the most stable in nature. This means that the body can be divided into four anterior quadrants and four posterior quadrants. Manaka went on to correlate these octants with the Eight Extraordinary Vessels (Eight Extras), and this core observation became the basis of his whole structural treatment approach. A discussion of these ideas, particularly how they relate to the Eight Extras, can be found in *Chasing the Dragon's Tail*. We return to Manaka's octahedron and the Eight Extras in more detail in chapter 12.

By extrapolating that the body is composed of four anterior and four posterior quadrants, Dr Manaka hypothesized a constantly interacting model, where the amount of qi flowing through each of the eight octants was regulated by the amount of qi flowing through the other seven. Thus, treatment aimed to restore the overall balance within the channel system between the inferior and superior, front and back, and left and right halves of the body. By regulating the channel system on the outside of the body, he could regulate the organ functioning on the inside of the body.

In fact, whatever your system of acupuncture or meridian-based bodywork, this is the essential yin-yang mechanism thought to be at work. We insert needles in the skin—the exterior—to affect the organs in the interior. With Ontake we don't insert needles; we simply warm the skin. Another difference is that with Ontake, we warm up broad areas of the skin, whereas we treat specific points with needles or small cone moxibustion. Later in this book, when we explore the uses of Ontake with different holographic systems, this difference will become very apparent. Instead of focusing on specific acupuncture points, Ontake "paints" broad areas with heat, rather like a painter and decorator using a roller instead of a fine brush.

Balloon Models

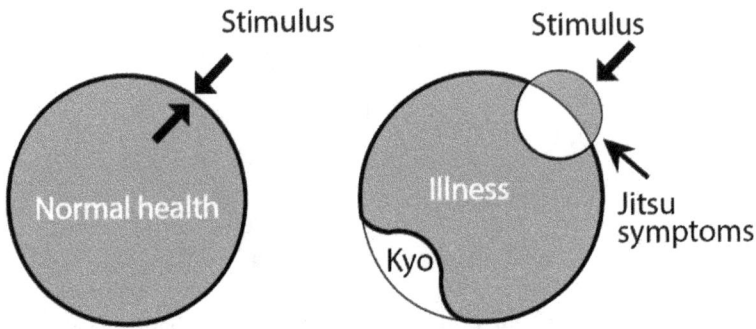

Dents and bumps: Masunaga's model of health and disease.

This idea of balancing qi flow to cure disease is not unique to Dr Manaka; it almost universal in TEAM, including in meridian-based bodywork methods such as Shiatsu. For example, renowned Japanese Shiatsu practitioner Shizuto Masunaga (1925–1981) described a balloon model. When someone is ill, it's as if an inflated balloon (the energy system) develops a dent (*kyo*, or "deficiency"). This dent is mirrored by a corresponding bump elsewhere in the system (*jitsu*, or "excess"). The purpose of treatment is to "iron out" these dents and bumps.[18]

A carpenter's contour gauge is another way of visualising these inner/outer relationships. Designed like a very dense comb but with moveable pins, you can press it against an irregular surface. The pressure depresses the pins at the points of contact on the inner facing edge and pushes them out at the outer facing edge, so they protrude symmetrically.

---

18   Matsunaga, S., & Ohashi, W. (2001). *Zen Shiatsu: How to Harmonize Yin and Yang for Better Health.* Tokyo: Japan Publications.

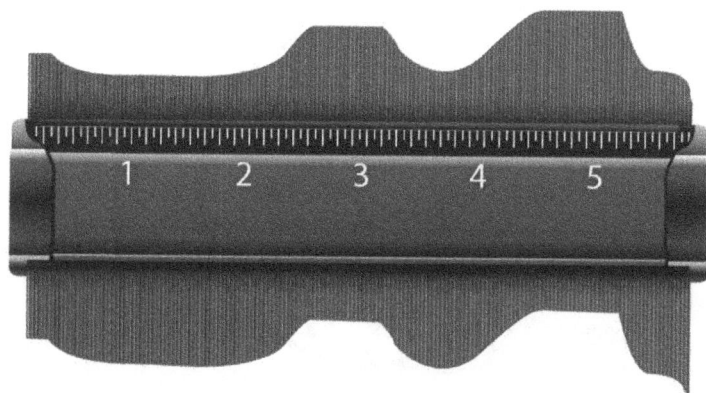

The contour gauge does in two dimensions what
Masunaga's balloon model does in three.

We can, however, see this process at work in the three-dimensional structure of the body with, for example, the lumbar curvature. If the lumbar curvature is too pronounced, as in anterior pelvic tilt, then the belly seems to protrude, even if the person is not overweight.

In other TEAM models, there are two concentric spheres. The inner sphere represents the *zangfu* organs, and the outer sphere represents the channels on the exterior of the body. If you depress or distort the outer sphere, like pressing on a balloon, corresponding protrusions may occur on the opposite side and the inner sphere. These distortions affect the functioning of the inner sphere. If you can correct the imbalances on the outside, you can improve the functioning of the organs on the inside.[19]

The concentric circles model has been progressively developed by Matsumoto and Birch in *Hara Diagnosis,* Birch and Felt in *Understanding Acupuncture,* and Birch in *Shonishin: Japanese Pediatric Acupuncture.*

19   Birch, S., & Felt, R. (1999). *Understanding Acupuncture.* Edinburgh: Churchill Livingstone, p.117; Matsumoto, K., & Birch, S. (1988). *Hara Diagnosis: Reflections on the Sea.* Brookline: Paradigm Publications, p. 234.

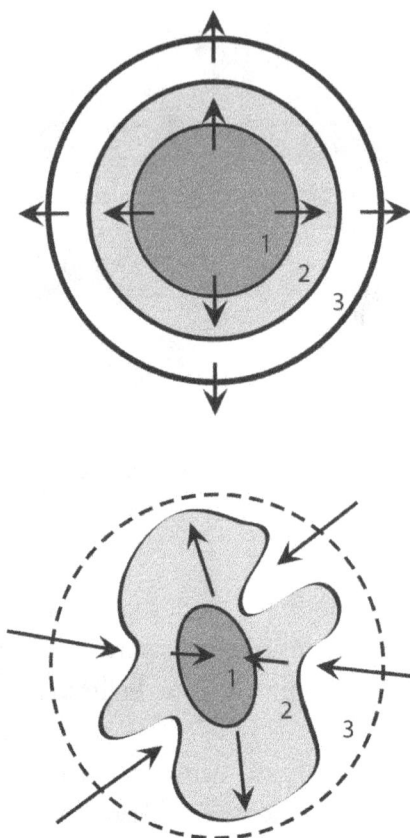

Birch model: 1. *Zangfu* Organs, 2. Channel Systems, 3. Overall Vitality.

In this model, the inner circle represents the *zangfu* organs and the functional systems of the body. The middle circle represents the channel systems, and the outer circle represents the overall vitality of the patient.

The second diagram shows how dents and bumps in the channel system, *kyo* and *jitsu* (deficiency and excess) can affect the functioning of the organs and the overall vitality of a person. Treatment is aimed at balancing *kyo* and *jitsu* in the channels so the functional systems can be repaired.[20]

These models are excellent ways to represent the fundamental relationships between yin and yang; interior and exterior; and structure and function and will inform our thinking about applying bamboo. These concepts need not be intellectual abstractions. The more you palpate the channels, the more you start to find remarkable parity between dents in one place and bumps in another.

After applying Ontake on one surface of the body, you will see immediate changes on an opposite surface. These surface shifts are reflections of systemic

---

20   Birch, S. (2016). *Shonishin Japanese Pediatric Acupuncture*. Stuttgart: Thieme, p. 56.

changes throughout the body, with significant knock-on changes taking place in the functional systems of the body and the overall vitality of our patients.

Kyo and Jitsu

Kyo and *jitsu*, discussed in Chinese as *xu* and *shi* and in some English texts either as deficiency and excess or as vacuity and repletion, have been widely explained in textbooks in column graphs representing different levels of yin and yang. Those levels rise and fall in relation to each other and within the context of a channel or organ. They denote a "relative measure of the shortage or surplus of a certain quality or quantity".[21]

Kyo (Deficiency)

Denmei Shudo, a renowned practitioner and teacher of Meridian Therapy in Japan, defines deficiency as "a lack of normal Qi in the organs, meridians or particular areas of the body".[22] There is a decline in vitality and physiological function, either overall or in a particular organ, channel, or area. This can be experienced through palpation as a feeling of emptiness, for example, as found in the flabby muscles of an eighty-year-old's arms.

Jitsu (Excess)

Excess is defined in two ways, first as an "abundance of pathogenic Qi".[23] Shudo explains that excess is a "state of increased activity in which the normal Qi of the body reacts to a pathogenic influence to produce a hyperactive condition in certain organs or meridians".[24] For example, when I am infected by a virus, my body mounts a fever in response.

A second kind of excess can be in response to a deficiency in the interior. It is this kind of excess in particular that is of interest to Ontake practice. As Ikeda notes, "When there is deficiency in one part of the body, another [organ or meridian] will increase in activity to compensate".[25]

---

21 Shudo, D. (1990). *Japanese Classical Acupuncture: Introduction to Meridian Therapy*. Seattle: Eastland Press, p. 30.

22 Ibid., p. 29.

23 Ibid., p. 29.

24 Ibid., p. 30.

25 Ikeda, M., *Zukai Shinkyu Igaku Nyumon,* quoted in Shudo, D. (1990). *Japanese Classical Acupuncture: Introduction to Meridian Therapy*. Seattle: Eastland Press, p. 30.

In addition to this, different categories of channels tend towards excess or deficiency: "yin organs and meridians have a tendency to become deficient, and yang organs and meridians to develop excessive conditions".[26] These are the dents and bumps discussed by Matsunaga and Birch. Structurally, this kind of deficiency and excess can be found in many places—for example, when a patient has cold feet, a red face, and tight shoulders (deficiency below, excess above).

The assessment of yin, yang, qi, blood, *kyo*, and *jitsu* may be the most challenging skill to learn in acupuncture treatment. Most traditional styles of acupuncture use the Four Examinations (Looking, Listening and Smelling, Asking, and Palpation) to arrive at this assessment, but there is considerable variation in the importance different styles put on different parts of the process.

Palpation is surprisingly overlooked in many acupuncture styles. However, in Meridian Therapy, there is a strong emphasis on palpation, not just of the pulse, but also on the *hara* (the abdomen) and the channels themselves. In Ontake treatment, deficiency and excess in the channels should be noted through visual observation and palpation, particularly by stroking and pressing along the channel pathways.

Though applying bamboo treatment is simple and easy to learn, choosing how and where to apply it takes more skill. Palpation is very important in this regard, and we return to it throughout the book.

Supplementing and Draining

Kodo Fukushima, the founder of the Toyohari Association of Japan, an organisation for blind acupuncturists, defined acupuncture as "the differentiation of *kyo* and *jitsu* followed by the application of *ho* and *sha*".[27]

As we have seen above, when there is deficiency, the "life supporting *ki* is depleted", so the needle technique needs to replenish this deficiency.[28] "When disease-related *ki* is in excess", the needle technique needs to remove disease related *ki* from the body. I often explain this idea to patients by comparing our role to that of Robin Hood. We steal from the rich to give to the poor. We divert energy from where there is much to where there is little.

---

26   Shudo, D. (1990). *Japanese Classical Acupuncture: Introduction to Meridian Therapy*. Seattle: Eastland Press, p. 108

27   Fukushima, K. (1991). *Meridian Therapy*. Tokyo: Toyo Hari Medical Association, p. 148.

28   Ibid.

The application of moxibustion for *ho* and *sha* is not as formalised as it is for needling. Generally, the application of slow and gentle heat is considered *ho*, and more rapid or hotter heat cycles are considered *sha*.[29]

Ontake is a subtle tool and versatile enough to allow techniques that supplement energy in the body or drain it. Generally speaking, superficial, gentle techniques with very light pressure on the skin are supplementing, and deeper, firmer techniques with more percussive strokes are more moving or draining.

Later we will look at how different techniques can achieve these two goals.

Regulation—"Acupuncture Doesn't Cure Anything"

The goal of meridian-based hari *therapy is the regulation of* ki *and* ketsu *[qi and blood]. Therefore, in this form of medicine, illness is seen as disturbances in the ki and ketsu, while health is recognized as their balance.*

—Kodo Fukushima[30]

Patients often ask if there is an acupuncture point for a specific symptom. "Can you do a point for knee pain? Is there a point for headaches? Which point should I press for sleep?" In some ways, and at certain levels, the answer to this is yes: there are acupuncture points for specific symptoms. P 6 is good for nausea, LIV 3 is good for headaches, and LI 1 is good for toothache.

This is also true of the Eight Extras. Their original uses were to treat symptoms. For shortness of breath, we should needle the master and coupled points of the Ren Mai (Conception Vessel). We can call this symptomatic acupuncture, and this approach certainly has an important role in treatment.

Traditional acupuncture, however, is not just about needling the right point for a specific symptom. The implication of the models above is that by adjusting the body back to its natural configuration, we improve its overall functioning. In other words, acupuncture does not "cure" anything: instead, it signals the body to cure itself. We send a signal from the outside of the body to the inside, and this signal triggers mechanisms in the body that create shifts in body function and levels of pain.

---

29   Ibid., p. 163.
30   Ibid., p. 37.

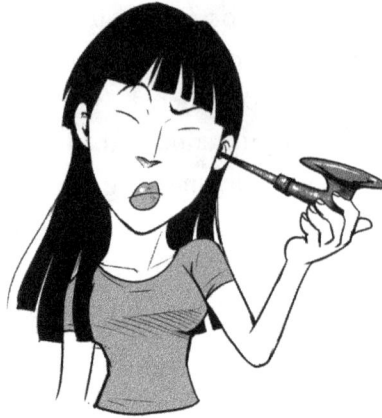

Acupuncture doesn't cure anything: instead,
it sends a signal that opens the door.

We can use the analogy of going to visit a favourite relative. When you arrive outside the house, you ring the doorbell. Eventually, the door opens, and Grandma emerges to greet you. We can all agree that it was not the doorbell that opened the door: it merely sent a signal to the interior of the house, and that signal created movement within it.

The Qi Paradigm

This signalling process is a core principle of traditional acupuncture, the so-called Qi Paradigm. The Qi Paradigm includes all traditional explanations for the mechanisms of acupuncture that refer to the Chinese concept of qi, often translated as "energy". Manaka had an alternative name for qi, namely the "X-signal system". This term suggests meanings that are not present in the word "energy". If we can think of qi as information and the channel system as an information highway, conveying signals, then we may gain a clearer understanding:

> There is a primitive signal (information) system in the body that has embryological roots, but is masked by the more advanced and complex control (regulation) systems. Thus, the original signal system is hard to find or see. This primitive system is able to detect and discriminate internal and external changes and plays a role in regulating the body by transmitting this information. This system serves as the modus operandi of acupuncture.[31]

---

31   Manaka, Y., Itaya, K., & Birch, S. (1995). *Chasing the Dragon's Tail: The Theory and Practice of Acupuncture in the Work of Yoshio Manaka.* Brookline: Paradigm Publications, p.18.

What's more, if we go back to the analogy of a doorbell, a doorbell typically uses minimal electrical current. While the results of ringing a doorbell may be dynamic, such as a teenager bounding noisily down the stairs to open the door, the doorbell remains a low-energy signalling system. Manaka had the same view of the channel system. It remains a very low-energy signalling system, and therefore, to access it, very low-energy stimulation is appropriate.

Thus, our role is not to do "stuff" to the body to cure a symptom ("stuff" is one of Stephen Birch's favourite humorous technical terms); our role is to signal, trigger or induce changes in the body when it is imbalanced so that it can find its own way to right itself. In traditional acupuncture, this process of signalling is the regulation of qi and blood. Many practitioners in Japan say that this is all an acupuncturist does: in daily practice, our role is simply to regulate qi and blood. Ontake is a tool that helps us to do this.

Ki and *Ketsu*

Another yin-yang pair worth considering in the context of Ontake is qi and blood, or *ki* and *ketsu*. *Ki* and *ketsu* circulate everywhere in the body, "bringing nutrition… fuelling growth and… combating disease.[32] Fukushima describes how *ying* qi and *wei* qi together (*ei-ketsu* and *e-ki*) circulate through the channels in the sequence of the Chinese clock:

"Ki is Yang… We know it by its actions but cannot make out its form. It flows on the outside of the meridians, accompanying and protecting the *ketsu.*"[33]

"*Ketsu* is Yin. It has form and flows, like the body fluids and blood, and moves on the inside of the meridians."[34]

Qi belongs to yang and has a warming function, while blood belongs to yin and has a nourishing function. Qi is said to be the commander of blood, and blood is the mother of qi. This means that where the qi leads, the blood follows. Thus, when we apply heat, vibration, and movement with bamboo on the skin, we are affecting the movement of qi on the exterior and the movement of blood in the interior.

Qi is light and insubstantial. Blood is material and has form. Qi is on the exterior, and blood is in the interior. This contrast between these concepts also implies a difference in the depth and seriousness of the disease. In Japanese acupuncture, problems can be seen at the qi level, which is more superficial, or the blood level,

---

32   Fukushima, K., (1991). *Meridian Therapy*. Tokyo: Toyo Hari Medical Association, p. 37.
33   Ibid.
34   Ibid.

which is deeper. The presentation of a symptom—for example, chest pain that comes and goes compared to chest pain that is fixed and constant—can tell you much about the level.

In other words, when a problem is at the qi level, it is less severe than when it progresses to the blood level. In some ways, this is just another way of saying acute and chronic, but in other ways, this is a way of understanding the depth and the seriousness of a disease.

Problems at the blood level are harder to treat and require a different approach to problems in the qi. For example, moxibustion is indicated when acupuncture is not effective because of its effect on the blood. Needles work more on qi—moxa more on blood. Shiraku (bloodletting) is indicated for stubborn and chronic problems which have not responded to conventional acupuncture and moxibustion treatment when there are clear signs of blood stasis.[35] Thus, for all chronic diseases, moxibustion is required. From this model, we can see that Bamboo is useful for chronic disease.

Root and Branch

> *The root treatment is more general. I say it is a "ground levelling". You know, if you have some rough ground then you have to make it flat. Then you will find some important part, some important point to dig to find something, so my idea is first just ground levelling, and then I find a good, good point to dig deeper and deeper and get some treasure from there. That's my idea of branch treatment. So, it varies. Two steps: the first step—just general treatment then the second step, you focus on the very important point.*

—Junji Mizutani[36]

The final yin-yang pairing to consider is the distinction made between the causes of a disease and the manifestations or symptoms of that disease. This means that acupuncture treatment can be categorised into two primary modes of action: root treatment (*honchiho*) and branch treatment (*hyochiho*).

---

35   Birch, S., & Ida, J. (1998) *Japanese Acupuncture: A Clinical Guide.* Brookline: Paradigm Publications, p. 212.

36   Mizutani, J. (2018, May 30). Interview by Oran Kivity with Stephen Birch, Junji Mizutani, and Brenda Loew. Retrieved from https://youtu.be/aoN3bwXmacY

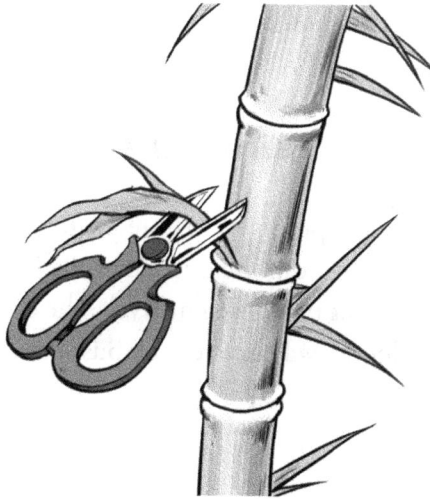

Branch treatment targets the symptoms, not the cause.

If you have a tall house plant with wilting or brown leaves, you can use a pair of scissors to cut them off. This makes the plant look better, but it doesn't fix the problem. If you take the opposite path—watering the roots to heal the plant—it takes much longer for the plant to recover fully. Treating the root means treating the underlying causes of the disease and treating the branch means treating the symptoms. Fukushima describes these two processes as fundamental healing and targeted healing.[37]

Some combination of root and branch treatment is necessary for effective outcomes. In acupuncture, there are purist schools that focus wholly on root treatment, and there are pragmatic approaches that focus wholly on branch treatment. Sadly, much current acupuncture research pays little attention to or misunderstands root and branch theory.[38] This research bias fails to understand the importance of these two different approaches.

What little has been published about treatment with bamboo ring moxa shows that it has been used mostly as an adjunctive branch treatment, an additional layer of symptomatic treatment to help resolve a problem.

As has been seen above, in Japanese acupuncture, the primary role of the practitioner is seen to be the regulation of *ki, ketsu, kyo*, and *jitsu*. Assessing the condition of *kyo* and *jitsu* is both the most difficult and the most important task facing us. Treatment with Ontake is no different, and the premise is the same. If we

---

37   Fukushima, K., (1991). *Meridian Therapy*. Tokyo: Toyo Hari Medical Association, p.37.
38   Birch, S. (2018, May 30). Interview by Oran Kivity with Stephen Birch, Junji Mizutani, and Brenda Loew. Retrieved from https://youtu.be/aoN3bwXmacY

regulate the flow of *ki* and *ketsu* and balance *kyo* and *jitsu* in the channels, the body will regulate itself.

Summary

Ontake can be used to treat symptoms or help regulate the body system as a whole. Like a doorbell, it sends a signal from the outside to the inside, triggering changes.

Health problems can exist at two different levels, the qi level and the blood level. Chronic problems at the blood level require moxibustion.

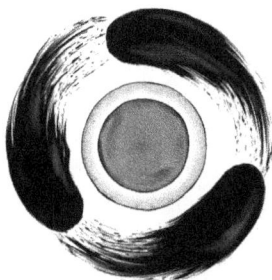

CHAPTER 4

TAPPING ZONES

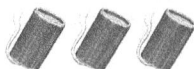

Introducing Manaka's meridian frequencies, mapping them on
the body, and offering principles to decide which frequencies to
use in areas where many channels are crowded together.

---

*What is important is the need for, and utilization of, a creative and consistent
research methodology and methods of assessing the effects of treatment. We can take
nothing at face value because without clinical tests and confirmation, we have no
real idea of what these simplifications mean.*

—*Yoshio Manaka*[39]

Manaka and the *Mu* Points

As we have seen before, Dr Manaka had a magpie mind. If he heard of a shiny new
idea, he was drawn to it. Importantly, he was also meticulously research oriented,
continuously testing new ideas, integrating what worked and discarding what did

---

39   Manaka, Y., Itaya, K., & Birch, S. (1995). *Chasing the Dragon's Tail: The Theory and Practice
of Acupuncture in the Work of Yoshio Manaka*. Brookline: Paradigm Publications, p. 12.

not. As Stephen Birch tells the story, a story that he himself was told, Dr Manaka was walking past a music shop with a group of students when something in the window caught his eye. He disappeared inside and reappeared carrying a metronome under one arm. "Let's find out which frequencies the meridians respond to!" he allegedly said.

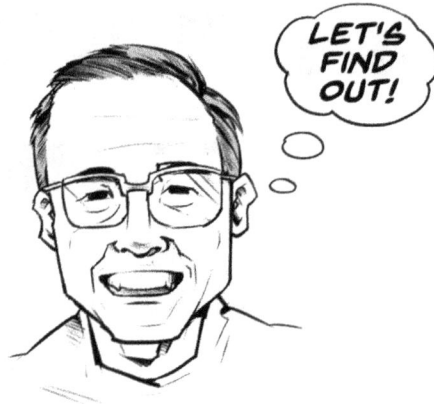

Dr Manaka experimented with sounds, frequencies, and pulsed magnetic fields.

Mythical or not—and we must assume that as the story has been told and retold, there is a core of truth and a coating of good-humoured elastic—this story illustrates a classic dilemma of acupuncture research. Even if you have a question, you need to find a tool with which to answer it. Even if you dare to imagine that the meridians can respond to frequencies, how can you design a test that distinguishes the frequencies of each?

To devise a test, Dr Manaka had already turned, in part at least, to the classics. In classical acupuncture, there is a group of twelve points called the front-*mu* ("alarm") points, all distributed on the chest or abdomen. Each point is said to be infused with the energy of its respective organ.

The term '*mu*' means "to gather or collect, and the front-*mu* points are where the qi of the zangfu gathers and concentrates on the anterior surface of the body".[40]

As "Yang diseases travel through the Yin region", these points "manifest signs such as stiffness and bumps during Yang illnesses".[41] The stiffness and bumps cause pain on palpation, and this pressure pain is used diagnostically.

---

40   Deadman, P., Al-Khafaji M., Baker K., (1998). *A Manual of Acupuncture*, East Sussex, England, : Journal of Chinese Medicine Publications. p. 44.

41   Fukushima, K., (1991). *Meridian Therapy*. Tokyo: Toyo Hari Medical Association, p. 173.

Thus, although the uses of front-*mu* points include treating related organs directly or treating local problems on the anterior, Dr Manaka was most attracted to how they could be used diagnostically. When there is a problem in with a front-*mu* point channel, it becomes tender on palpation. When the problem is treated, the tenderness disappears.

The twelve classical front-*mu* points are all located on the chest and abdomen, close to their related organs. LU 1, LIV 14 and GB 24 are the front-*mu* points for lung, liver and gall bladder organs, respectively, but the other nine front-*mu* points are not on their related channel. Interestingly, the front-*mu* points for pericardium, heart, stomach, triple burner and small intestine are all on the midline, at REN 17, REN 14, REN 12, REN 5 and REN 4, respectively.

As Dr Manaka's octahedral model is very concerned with, among other things, assessing left and right balances, he felt that these classical midline points were not able to give him the feedback he needed. You can easily detect differences between LU 1 on the right and on the left that reflect the condition of the right and left lung channels. However, if you palpate REN 12, the front-*mu* point of the stomach, which is on the midline, you have no way to differentiate the left stomach channel from the right.

To overcome this problem, in the course of developing his octahedral model, Dr Manaka researched and identified other points that get reactive but are located bilaterally. In the example above, he palpated laterally to REN 12 in a horizontal line connecting both ST 21 points. This solution was the origin of the Manaka Mu Points, a set of twelve diagnostic points with several key properties essential to Dr Manaka's research and clinical work:

1. Just like the classical *mu* points, when there are problems in the related channel, the Manaka Mu Points feel tight or painful on palpation.
2. This tightness or pain changes swiftly when the channel is treated.
3. The Manaka Mu Points are not on the midline, so each pair can be used to differentiate left and right channel flow.

These points are presented and discussed in *Chasing the Dragon's Tail* and are an essential component of practising MSA. What the humorous music shop story above suggests is that Dr Manaka suddenly got the idea to research meridian frequencies when his eye alighted on a metronome in a shop window. This, of course, is not really what happened. All great discoveries and inventions are on a continuum, where one question or experiment leads to another, which leads to another.

Frequencies

We have already used the analogy of a doorbell for acupuncture. It sends a signal from the outside of the house to the inside, creating movement when someone comes to answer the door. Rather than calling this signal "qi", Dr Manaka tried to understand qi as an information system, what he called the X-signal system. How does the body transmit information during acupuncture? He was already familiar with point location tools that measure skin resistance. As the channel system demonstrated specific characteristics, such as being electrically measurable, could there be a relationship between the channels and different frequencies? Equipped with his own set of dynamic reflex points, Dr Manaka experimented with sounds, frequencies, and pulsed magnetic fields:

> Using an oscilloscope with headphones, we found that playing sounds to a subject in the low-frequency range (50 Hz) reduced pressure pain and tension along the abdominal midline. Sounds in the higher frequency range (1000 Hz) reduced pressure pain and tension at the lateral edges of the abdomen, even in subjects with very stubborn reactions. Curiously, in schizophrenics, the reverse was true.[42]

When using pulsed magnetic fields, he observed the same thing: "We subjected different acupoints on the limbs to low and high frequency pulsed electromagnetic fields...low frequency affected the midline of the body; high frequency affected the lateral edges".[43]

Maybe it was at this point in his research that Dr Manaka's roving eye spotted the metronome in the shop window.

> In order to investigate frequency relationships for each of the channels, we adopted another approach. Using a SEIKO quartz metronome, which emits regular clicks at a rate of 40 to 208 clicks per minute, we recorded the frequency that appeared to affect each of the twelve main channels and the *ren mai* and *du mai* by reducing pressure pain and tightness at related reflex points and areas ... We set the metronome at different rates, letting the subject listen to the clicks while we repalpated the reactive acupoints.[44]

---

42   Manaka, Y., Itaya, K., & Birch, S. (1995). *Chasing the Dragon's Tail: The Theory and Practice of Acupuncture in the Work of Yoshio Manaka*. Brookline: Paradigm Publications, p. 71.

43   Ibid, p. 71.

44   Ibid, p. 71.

We can imagine this process took considerable time, with Manaka working first with colleagues and students, then with patients in his hospital. Eventually "using this method of investigation on many subjects", he was able to create a table of channel frequency correspondences.

Table 2 Meridian Frequencies Grouped by Channel

Yang	Frequency (beats per minute)	Yin	Frequency (beats per minute)
GB	120	LIV	108
SI	120	HT	126
ST	132	SP	132
LI	108	LU	126
BL	112	KID	120
TB	152	P	176
DU MAI	104	REN MAI	104

Having established this table, he then went on to test the frequencies in clinical practice. Here is an example:

> We used this method on a patient with pain in the left leg, difficulty walking and pressure pain and tension along the stomach, gall bladder and bladder channels of the left leg below the knee. Tapping GV 14, the intersection *jiaohui* point for all the yang channels, alternately at a rate of 132 beats (stomach), then 120 beats (gall bladder), and 112 beats (bladder) per minute, for twenty taps per rate, consecutively reduced the pressure pain and tension along the stomach, gall bladder and bladder channels. The patient's pain was much reduced, and the patient experienced greater ease when walking. These and numerous other clinical examples provide confirmation of these channel frequency-correspondences.[45]

Since writing this in the late 1980s, Dr Manaka's method has been taught extensively around the world and has continued to be used by many practitioners. It was the extraordinary efficacy of these meridian frequency correlations with the

---

45   Ibid. p. 72.

wooden needle and hammer that led me to start applying them first with a moxa stick and then with Ontake.

Looking at the table above, we can see that several channels share frequencies. Here are the same fourteen channels arranged by frequency, from low to high.

Table 3 Channels Grouped by Frequency

Frequency	Channels
104	DU, REN
108	LI, LIV
112	BL
120	KID, SI, GB
126	HT, LU
132	ST, SP
152	TB
176	P

Tapping with Bamboo

If you know your channel pathways, tapping with the wooden hammer or Ontake is a simple matter. If you are on the lung channel, for example, tap at 126 beats per minute. If you are on the large intestine channel, tap at 108. It's that simple.

Manaka's wooden hammer had one principal method of application—tapping—but there are many ways to apply bamboo, including tapping, rolling, pressing, vibrating, and bouncing. Rather than using the term "apply bamboo", I use the word "tap" as a generic term that encompasses all these methods of application. Patients in my practice like the word "bamboozle"!

As this book is aimed at practitioners who have prior knowledge of the qi paradigm and the channel pathways, there seems little point in reproducing the channel pathway information already presented in many acupuncture textbooks. The information I have used comes from the excellent *Manual of Acupuncture* by Peter Deadman et al.[46]

---

46   Deadman, P., Al-Khafaji, M., & Baker, K., (1998). *A Manual of Acupuncture*. East Sussex, England: Journal of Chinese Medicine Publications, p. 44.

Mapping the Frequency Zones

If we take the information in Table 2 and colour a diagram of the body by frequency instead of by channel, we can map the meridian frequencies and develop a composite picture of the tapping zones. For the most part, what I present here follows the standard meridian pathways and the frequencies presented by Dr Manaka, with some pragmatic exceptions.

When working on any area with a known channel pathway, for example from LU 5 to LU 9, it is simple to apply the appropriate frequency. But in certain areas, the channel pathways are more intricate, so it has made more sense to generalise. Mapping the tapping zones is a continual work in progress, a synthesis of channel pathways, channel frequencies, and pragmatic and empirical decisions made after extended practice. This is because there are differences between tapping with a wooden needle and hammer on a point and rolling over a broad area with Ontake. We need to make a clear distinction between treating areas and channels.

For example, if specifically working on KID 25 to KID 27 on the chest, we should tap at kidney frequency (120). In some instances, however, you may want to tap on the whole anterior upper right torso: this includes Ren Mai, stomach, kidney, lung, pericardium, spleen, heart, and even gall bladder channels. Rather than continually changing frequency by channel, the aim is to warm a whole area, and in these cases, I use a generic frequency. In this example, I use 126 beats per minute, the frequency of lung and heart, which comprise the upper burner. Of course, this can be done using no frequency at all, but as will be seen in later discussions, the sound of the metronome gives a structure and predictability to treatment that should not be underestimated.

Thus, the principles for frequency selection are:
- When treating points, use the channel frequency.
- When treating channels, use the channel frequency.
- When treating large areas that encompass several channels, use a generic frequency, related to the area in TEAM theory. This includes sense organs such as the eyes, ears, and nose.

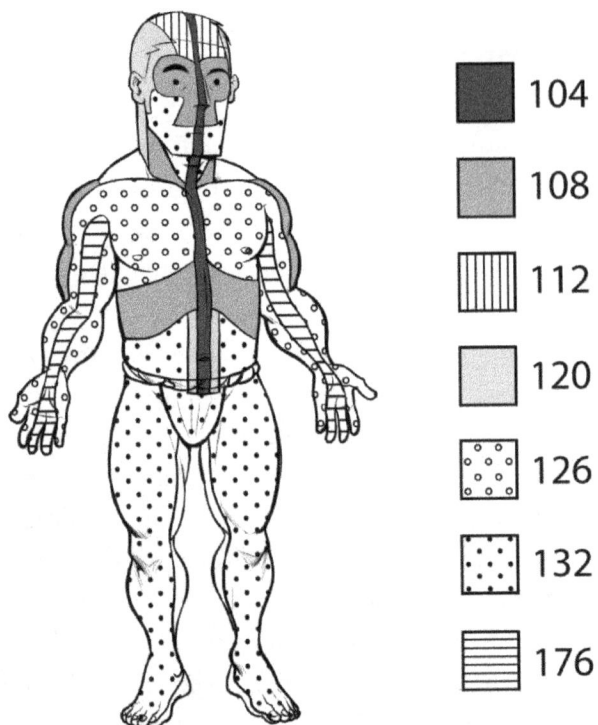

■	104
▨	108
▥	112
▢	120
▦	126
⋰	132
☰	176

Tapping zones: anterior view.

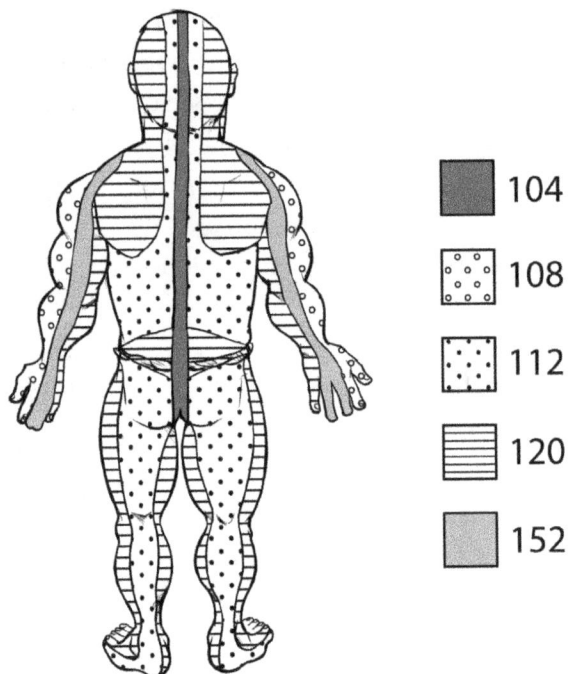

■	104
▦	108
⋰	112
☰	120
▨	152

Tapping zones: posterior view.

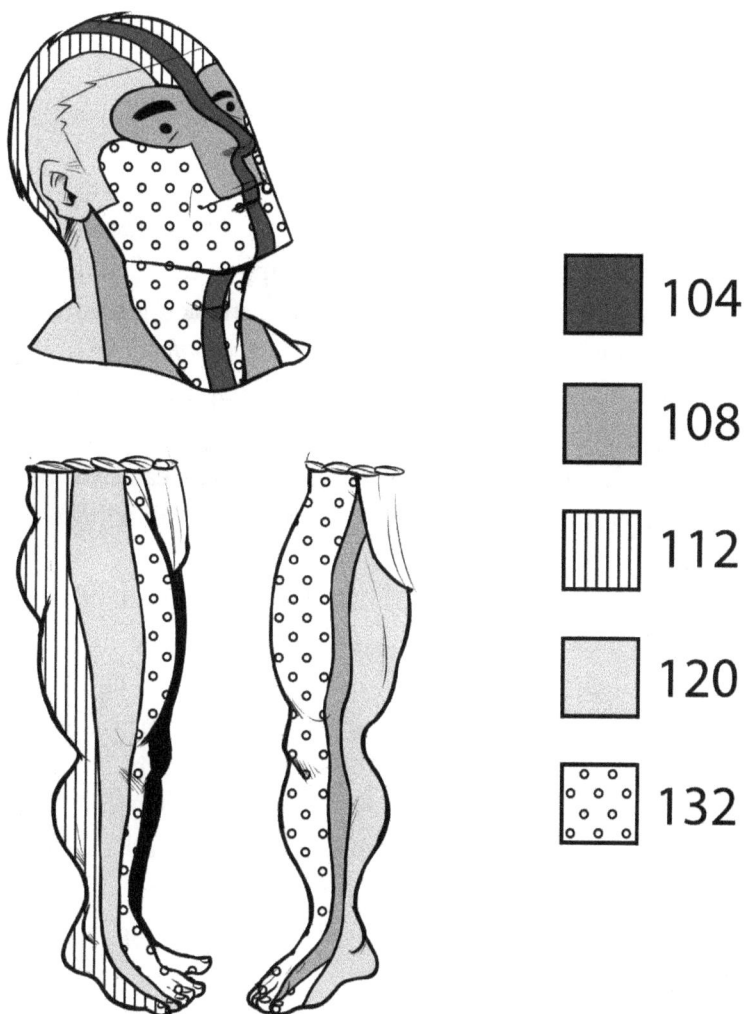

Tapping zones: head and leg.

As we view the channel frequencies in this way, we can see in very general terms that Manaka's observation that low-frequency sounds affect the midline and high-frequency sounds affect the lateral aspect of the abdomen seems to be correct as a general rule for meridian tapping, but there are some exceptions.

On the midline of the posterior trunk, Du Mai reacts to the lowest frequency (104). As you move more laterally, you encounter bladder (112), small intestine (120), and gall bladder in the axilla (120).

On the midline of the anterior trunk, Ren Mai reacts to the lowest frequency (104). As you move out from kidney (120) to stomach (132) and spleen (132), the frequencies get higher, yet the gall bladder, at the most lateral aspect of the trunk, has a frequency (120) that is lower than that of stomach and spleen.

Pragmatic Tapping

Back

The back is an area of crucial importance that you will find yourself treating frequently. There are many reasons for this. Firstly, the back is a holographic microsystem of the whole body. The back-*shu* points reflect the upper, middle, and lower parts of the body on a one-to-one scale.[47] For this reason, many acupuncture traditions and methods emphasise the importance of treating the back-*shu* points. When treating children with Shonishin, we rub both sides of the spine from top to bottom.[48] Chinese texts cite systemic treatments with the plum blossom needle, treating both sides of the spine.[49] Ontake treatment is no different. You can treat the whole back and back of the legs in a few minutes and get system-wide effects. Most importantly, patients love bamboo on the back.

As we have seen, the lowest frequency Du Mai (104) is in the centre. The bladder channel covers most of the back, so the most common frequency to use when treating the back is 112.

As gall bladder and small intestine channels share the same frequency, the lateral aspect of the back, the scapula, and the top of the shoulders can all be treated at 120 beats per minute. Thus, you can effectively cover the whole back with two frequencies: 112 and 120, adding 104 if working directly on the spine.

Occasionally, the top of the trapezius around GB 21 and TB 15 remains very tight after treating at 120. In these cases, it is worth palpating again and changing frequency to 152, to release triple burner.

When treating acute tightness in the lower back, it is sometimes useful to switch to 120 beats per minute. Perhaps this is because the gall bladder sinew channel traverses this area. This is marked as an optional rhomboid shape on the lower back, where you can also tap at 120 beats per minute. The area around GB26 on the lateral aspect of the abdomen should also be tapped at 120 beats per minute and is useful for releasing the neck. This relationship between the neck and the waist, *kubi koshi* in Japanese, is explored in detail in chapter 12.

---

47   Dale, R. (1999). The Systems, Holograms and Theory of Micro-Acupuncture *American Journal of Acupuncture, 27*(3-4), 207–42.

48   Birch, S. (2016). *Shonishin Japanese Pediatric Acupuncture*. Stuttgart: Thieme, p.48.

49   Auteroche, B. (1998). *Acupuncture and Moxibustion: A Guide to Clinical Practice*. Edinburgh: Churchill Livingstone.

Back of the Legs

If you have finished with the back, you might want to continue down the legs. This is very simple, as the bladder channel covers the posterior of the legs, allowing you to treat from buttock to ankle at 112 beats per minute. Treating the bladder channel in this way has distal effects from the head to the waist.

Side of the Legs

The gall bladder channel runs down the lateral part of the leg covering the tensor fascia lata (TFL). If working on lateral tension, such as a tight TFL or tight calf muscles, you can start once again at the glutes and work your way down the side of the legs at 120 beats per minute.

The gall bladder, small intestine and kidney channels share the same frequency, 120 beats per minute. On the thigh, the kidney channel is posteromedial, becoming slightly more medial on the calf. This means that when you get to the calf, there are two strips on either side, medial and lateral, that respond to 120 beats per minute.

Usually, in prone position, these two frequencies, 112 and 120 beats per minute, are all you need to release the buttocks, thighs, and calves. Tapping on kidney and gall bladder channels has distal effects on the neck, shoulder, and waist.

Front of the Legs

The stomach and spleen channels cover the anterior part of the legs. In the colour version of the diagram, the model looks like he is wearing a pair of yellow leggings. If required, it is a simple matter to treat the whole anterior leg at 132 beats per minute. This can be very useful for abdominal pain, epigastric pain, and stiff shoulders.

Liver Channel

In generalised bamboo treatments, I have not found it necessary to treat the liver channel to relax the whole leg, unless there are particularly tight points that need attention. The adjacent channels are more accessible. However, the liver channel is useful for treating specific conditions and symptoms, especially applying bamboo around LIV 3 to LIV 5. Stagnating pain in the lower abdomen or testicles responds well to this kind of treatment. Also, as we will see later in chapter 11, this area can be very effective for shoulder and neck pain in the small intestine channel.

I do not recommend rolling up and down the liver channel on the inner thigh, particularly with female patients, as this could be considered intrusive. However, when training in China, I saw doctors recommend that patients with dysmenorrhoea should roll their inner thighs with a baker's rolling pin to relieve their pain. This method can be adapted to bamboo, and patients respond very well to rolling bamboo on the liver channel at 108 beats per minute. The combination of applied warmth and frequency makes the relief much faster than with a rolling pin alone.

An alternative area for menstrual pain to roll is on the spleen channel between SP6 and SP8 at 132 beats per minute.

Chest and Ribcage

The heart channel originates in the armpit, and this can be a beneficial area to tap, particularly for gall bladder–type headaches (see chapter 11). The lung channel originates in the pectoral area, and this can be helpful to address lower back pain (see chapter 12). We can also tap the kidney channel at 120 beats per minute

If tapping on a single channel on the torso, select the frequency according to the channel. For heart and lung channels, tap at 126 beats per minute; for the kidney channel,120 beats per minute; for the stomach, 132 beats per minute; and for Ren Mai, 104 beats per minute. There are so many channels running through the chest, however, that it may feel disruptive to keep switching frequencies on your metronome. In this case, it is better to be pragmatic and treat at a generic frequency. As the upper burner contains the lung and heart organs, their shared frequency, 126, seems appropriate as a generic selection for the chest.

Interestingly the whole chest is covered by Hirata zones 1-3, relating to the bronchi, lungs, and heart. Hirata Zone Therapy is a holographic system for treatment developed in the early twentieth century and will be introduced later in the book. With this extra information, it makes even more sense to tap the chest at a generic 126 beats per minute.

The sides of the rib cage respond to 132 beats per minute (spleen) or 120 beats per minute (gall bladder). *Shidou* SP 17 is a bilateral point, but some sources refer to SP17 on the left side by another name, *Mingguan*. *Mingguan* has some quite esoteric indications for when "life is hanging by a thread" and can be used for any spleen disease.[50] Since the point is level with the apex of the heart, I have found it useful to tap here at 132 beats per minute for chest pain and to relieve anxiety.

Moving further down the ribcage and as far as the hypochondriac region, we need to make another pragmatic decision. Once again, knowledge of Hirata zones can help us. This is zone 4, which relates to the liver. As the hypochondriac region

---

50   Deadman, P., Al-Khafaji, M., & Baker, K., (1998). *A Manual of Acupuncture*. East Sussex, England: Journal of Chinese Medicine Publications, p. 202.

also reflects liver pathology in other acupuncture traditions, I generally tap above and below the costal margin at a generic liver frequency (108).

Abdomen

The abdomen is very simple to map. It is dominated by the stomach and spleen, both anatomically and functionally, so it seems logical to treat generically at 132 beats per minute. When working on the midline, use 104 beats per minute, and when working on kidney channel use 120 beats per minute. Tapping on the kidney channel in this region can be helpful for treating neck and back pain (see chapter 12).

Arms

The yang surface of the arm holds no surprises. Each channel—large intestine, triple burner, and small intestine—has its frequency and can be followed up into the shoulder.

The yin surface is more interesting because heart and lung channels share the same frequency, 126 beats per minute. Thus, the yin surface has two tapping zones, medial and lateral, that require relatively low frequencies, and one tapping zone, the pericardium on the median line, with the highest frequency of all, 176 beats per minute.

It is interesting to note that both the leg and the arm have medial and lateral bands that respond to the same frequency: the kidney and gall bladder (120), and the heart and lungs (126).

Head and Face

Coming finally to the head, it is worth discussing whether we should do moxa in this area at all. Surely, if the head is yang and moxa is yang, we are asking for trouble by applying moxa here. This is not really the case.

Moxa is frequently given on the head, both in Chinese traditions, for example, moxa on DU 20 to raise spleen qi and treat prolapse,[51] and in Japanese traditions, such as *kyutoshin* (warm needle) at GB 20 for headache.[52] Hirata and Manaka, forty years apart, both wrote books describing procedures for applying a specialised heated needle on the Hirata zones on the head. Ontake, more warm than hot, has a subtle

---

51   Ibid. p. 553.
52   Birch, S., & Ida, J. (1998) *Japanese Acupuncture: A Clinical Guide.* Brookline: Paradigm Publications, p. 104.

warming effect on the skin. Rather than heating the body and "adding yang", it can be used for gentle supplementation, moving or draining techniques. Thus, moxa can be used on the head without fear. What we should consider, however, is that as the head is bony; it therefore requires a lighter kind of application than other parts of the body.

As on the back, we see the central line of the Du Mai (104) flanked on either side by the bladder channel (112) and the gall bladder (120). Triple burner encircles the ear (152). In TEAM, the ear belongs to the kidneys, so when working on ear issues, I tap gall bladder (120) in a broad circle around the ear, triple burner in a tighter circle (152), and the ear itself at a generic 120 beats per minute, the kidney frequency. Needless to say, the ear is such a powerful acupuncture microsystem that bamboo applied here feels extremely relaxing. Try it yourself!

When treating specific areas on the forehead, we can choose 104 beats per minute for the midline, 120 beats per minute for above the eyes, and 132 beats per minute for the lateral margins. If wanting to treat the whole forehead without constantly changing frequencies, it is easier to treat unaccompanied, without the metronome or by choosing a generic frequency—132 beats per minute, for example, as frontal headaches relate to stomach foot *yangming* channel.

Treating the midline from *Yintang* to Du 20 can bring quick relief for nasal congestion, allergies, and inflammation.

Many channels innervate the eye, but because the liver opens into the eye, I like to tap at a generic 108 beats per minute. In TEAM theory, the lungs open into the nose, so we can use a generic frequency of 126 beats per minute when tapping there. We can also think of the neighbouring influence of the large intestine channel and tap at 108 beats per minute, thus using one frequency for the eyes and nose.

The rest of the face can be said to belong mainly to stomach channel (132), and bamboo has immense benefits as an easily applied moxibustion tool in cases of facial paralysis and TMJ syndromes.

Neck

The neck is quite awkward to treat with frequencies because it is a smaller compact area where the channels run close together. As we will see later when discussing the Toyohari concepts of *naso muno*, treating the neck can have systemic effects on problems in the upper part of the body. Thus, we need to use channel or area rules to select the frequency. If you are working on one channel, such as stomach, then select the channel frequency. If you are working on the neck in broad strokes, then select a generic frequency, such as 120 beats per minute, that affects both the small intestine and gall bladder.

Table 4 Tapping Zones Summary

Head	Midline DU	104
	Lateral to midline BL	112
	Sides GB	120
Ear	Three circles around the ear GB TB Ear	 120 152 120 (generic for kidney)
Eye	Tap around the orbit	108 (generic for the eye)
Forehead	Whole *yangming* area	132
	Specific channels such as BL or GB	112, 120
Face	ST	132
Nose	LI LU	108 126 (generic for lung)
Neck Lateral Posterior	 SI/GB BL	 120 112
Chest	LU/HT	126 (generic)
Ribcage/ hypochondrium	LIV	108 (generic)
Abdomen	ST/SP Midline KID	132 104 120
Inguinal groove	GB and ST/SP	120/132
Back	Midline	104
	Sides of spine and lateral	112
	Trapezius	120/152
	Scapula	120
Lumbar region	BL	112
Waist	The area above GB 26 Alternative frequency for lumbar region	120 120

Upper limb	Yin aspect has parallel stripes at HT/LU, with P in the middle. Yang aspect follows three yang channels, LI, TB & SI.	126, 176 108, 152, 120
Lower limb	Anterior aspect ST/SP Posterior aspect: BL Lateral aspect: KID, GB	132 112 120

Intersection Points

Many points on the body are intersection points between two or more channels. Like a busy train station, many lines pass through a single point. The most notable of these is DU 14, which is the intersection point of seven channels: the six yang channels and the Du Mai itself. Other useful points are ST 12 and SP 6. Dr Manaka demonstrated that these points could be used as "wild cards", in that they respond to tapping at the frequency of any of the intersecting channels. For example, SP 6 can be tapped not just at spleen frequency but also at the frequency of liver and kidney. Treating multiple channels from one point in this way can have very useful clinical effects.

In terms of Ontake treatment, when treating pain on the yang channels, DU 14 is often used as a closing point, either by vibrating while scrolling down all the yang frequencies from 152 to 104 beats per minute or just rubbing at the frequency of the yang channel that was affected. For example, if someone has pain in the fourth finger on the triple burner channel, vibrating DU 14 at 152 beats per minute can be very helpful.

SP 6 can be used to treat peripheral neuropathy, scrolling through the frequencies of the three leg yin channels.

Meridian Pairings and the Effects of Bamboo

As is apparent from the observations above, bamboo can be used locally (where the pain is) and to generate systemic body-wide effects. Yin channels tend towards deficiency, and yang channels tend towards excess. Thus, working on paired channels can be very useful. A simple example of this is that when the kidney channel is weak, the bladder channel can get tight. By treating the deficiency on the kidney channel, you can rapidly relieve pain in the bladder channel. These pairings are the mainstay of Ontake's most spectacular effect—namely, the rapid relief of pain. We will explore these pairings in depth in chapter 11, adapting the work of Dr Richard Tan.

Summary

Dr Manaka's frequencies can be mapped out on the body using three principles: point theory, channel theory, and generalised TEAM theory. Tapping on a channel can have both local and distal effects. The intersection points can be used as wild cards, with tapping applied at the frequency of any of the intersecting channels.

Now that we have figured out the frequencies for each area of the body, what's next? What should we look for on each channel when we start to treat it? The next chapter introduces palpation and the perception of *kyo* and *jitsu*.

PART 2

ROOT AND BRANCH

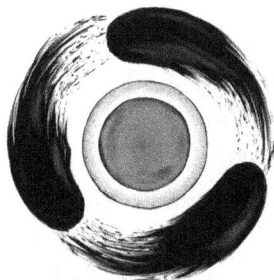

CHAPTER 5

KYO, JITSU, AND PALPATION

Introducing concepts important to palpation, such as the feel
of *kyo* and *jitsu*, and a routine for tension assessment.

---

*In diagnosis there are five areas that deserve close examination. They are the pulses,
the channels that correspond to the organs, the muscles, the tendons and the acupoints.
In general, close scrutiny of these five areas will provide sufficient information to
make a proper diagnosis.*

—*Nei Jing Su Wen* [53]

Kyo and *Jitsu*

In earlier pages, we explored *kyo and jitsu* in general terms as relative measures of
deficiency or excess of certain qualities. In traditional acupuncture styles, we arrive
at an overall assessment of deficiency and excess through the Four Examinations—

---

53   Ni, M. (1995). *The Yellow Emperors Classic of Medicine: A New Translation of the Neijing Suwen
with Commentary.* Boston, MA: Shambhala.

Looking, Listening and Smelling, Asking, and Palpation—leading to an identification of a pattern of deficiency-excess (*kyojitsu*) in channel or organ systems.

Different styles of acupuncture emphasise different aspects of this process of pattern recognition. In TCM, which emphasises the ingestion of herbs, the questioning with regard to organ function is very detailed. In Japanese acupuncture, however, there is less emphasis on asking and more on palpation—not just of the pulse, but of the abdomen and the channels themselves. The reasons for this have been explored by many authors, but the historically high numbers of blind acupuncturists in Japan are thought to have made the use of touch much more predominant as a diagnostic tool.[54] The significance of "abnormal tissue findings" found through palpation is a major theme in Japanese acupuncture generally.[55]

For this reason, in the Toyohari Association of Japan, which teaches a Meridian Therapy approach using Five Phase diagnosis, stroking the channels, particularly on the yin aspect of the forearm is part of the training and diagnostic routine. Even in China, where there had previously been little emphasis on channel palpation, there has been a small renaissance, spearheaded by the late Wang Ju Yi.[56]

The blind practitioners of the Toyohari Association often speak of the "lustre" of the skin. Lustre, of course, was originally a visual term. When speaking of the colour black, for example, we can compare the lustre of a raven's wing with the lustre of coal dust. A raven's wing has a sheen of life and vitality, whereas coal dust does not.

Evidently, the blind practitioners are not talking about the appearance of lustre, but its feel, the sensation under your fingers when you stroke the patient's skin. This feel of the skin is an essential diagnostic element in Toyohari, which can give you many clues about the patient's overall condition.

As Toyohari instructor Takashi Nakayama writes, "Lustre is not explained by warmth alone. It could also manifest as brightness, moisture, smoothness or springiness".[57] Skin with good lustre feels vibrant, warm, and smooth. Skin with poor lustre feels dry and rough. If we imagine stroking the skin of a grandparent and that of a teenager, we can immediately picture the feel of their respective lustres and how we could distinguish these two separate sensations. However, if this is true for

---

54   Birch, S., & Ida, J. (1998) *Japanese Acupuncture: A Clinical Guide.* Brookline: Paradigm Publications, p. 4.

55   Chant, B., Madison, J., Coop, P., & Dieberg, G. (2017). Beliefs and values in Japanese acupuncture: an ethnography of Japanese trained acupuncture practitioners in Japan. *Integrative Medicine Research,* 6(3), 260–268. http://doi.org/10.1016/j.imr.2017.07.001

56   Wang, J.Y., & Robertson, J.D. (2008). *Applied Channel Theory in Chinese Medicine.* Seattle: Eastland Press, Inc.

57   Nakayama, T. (2017). Hiesho-Oversensitivity to the Cold. *Keiraku Chiryo – International Toyohari News,* p. 25.

two people at such opposite ends of the vitality spectrum, it must also be true for people who are also very close. Now imagine the lustre of a healthy teenager and an unhealthy one. This is a much finer task of differentiation, but one no less important to perform.

To date, there is no system of pattern recognition in Ontake treatment. We do not identify syndromes such as kidney deficiency or liver excess. Ontake is mostly used as an adjunctive treatment and can be incorporated into any system of acupuncture as an additional modality to address symptoms. It achieves this effect by balancing deficiency-excess within a single channel or pair of channels. This kind of deficiency-excess assessment in the channels can be performed with almost no theory, through touch alone. In Ontake treatment, therefore, channel palpation is of primary importance.

When applying Ontake, the objective is to identify then balance *kyojitsu* in the channel. The techniques should be moderated according to the condition of the skin and muscles. This localised application will, however, create other important, systemic effects, as we will see in later chapters.

Palpation Methods for Channel Assessment

I've adapted three principal ways to palpate the channels for the assessment of Ontake treatment. These comprise:
- Stroking
- Picking up and squeezing
- Pressing

Stroking

You can stroke an area with your whole hand or just your fingertips. Simply stroke very lightly over the area and notice the lustre of the skin. Do some areas feel warm, vibrant, smooth and healthy? Do other areas feel rough, dry, moist, or lacking in vitality? As you pass your hand over the surface, you may also notice the tone of the underlying tissue. There may be tightness or flaccidity at a deeper level.

You can try this right now, on yourself. Try stroking your anterior forearm, from elbow to wrist. You can also stroke the sides and front of your neck, from jaw to breastbone. How is the lustre in these two places?

If you're feeling tired today, you may notice some roughness or moistness in one or both of these areas.

Picking Up and Squeezing

Picking up and squeezing is a useful technique to use on the limbs. If standing to one side of a supine patient, you can use both hands to pick up and squeeze the thigh and note tension in the gall bladder, stomach and spleen channels all the way down the leg. On the arm, you can note the tension in the triple burner, large intestine, and lung. It is useful to do this as a general tension assessment and also when deciding which channel pair might be implicated when treating pain (see chapter 11).

Pressing

Light pressing with the tips of the fingers or slightly deeper pressing with the palm can inform you about deeper chains of tension in the body. For example, try pressing lightly with the tips of the fingers down the sides of the calf muscle when the patient is prone, and note tight areas on the kidney, gall bladder, and bladder channels.

With the patient lying supine, press with one palm on the left shoulder and one on the right hip, then reverse to one palm on the right shoulder and one on the left hip. How do the shoulders and hips respond? Is one diagonal axis tighter than the other?

The Feel of *Kyo* and *Jitsu*

People often overthink *kyo* and *jitsu*, not just when palpating but also when conceptualising. In simple terms, an excess is when something is present, and a deficiency is when nothing is. If there's resistance to your palpation, there's something there. If there's no resistance, nothing is there.

Kyo-Deficient Areas

If deficient or *kyo*, the skin may be cool, loose, inelastic, and flaccid. The general lustre is poor. Excessive dryness or moistness are also signs of deficiency. These areas require supplementing techniques with bamboo, such as very light rolling or tapping techniques that just contact the surface of the skin.

Jitsu-Excess Areas

If excess or *jitsu*, the muscles feel hard and tight. The skin lustre may be either good or poor, but on superficial or deeper palpation there will be stiffness or hardness.

These areas require rolling with more pressure, tapping with a more percussive stroke, or pressing techniques with the lip or side of the bamboo. When these areas are stubborn, it is useful to think of distal areas and related channels. For example, the back of the calf affects the lumbar area, and the lung channel releases the lumbar area through its *shigo* (midday-midnight) polar channel pair relationship (see chapter 11).

Table 5 *Kyo* and *Jitsu*

Kyo	*Jitsu*
Depressed	Raised, elevated
Soft	Hard
Weak	Strong
Moist	
Cool/cold	Hot
Roughness, dryness	
Puffy	Swollen
Flabby/loose	Tight, stiff
Inelastic	
Underdeveloped	Overdeveloped
Insensitivity	Tenderness, pressure pain

Pressure pain

The late Katsuo Tsuboi was a senior instructor in the Toyohari Association. Like most blind practitioners, his palpatory skills were very refined. He observed that in some areas, palpation felt good to some patients but uncomfortable to others. Sometimes sensations vary according to depth, and these findings can inform our understanding of *kyojitsu*.

Table 6 Deficient or Excess Pain[58]

Kyo pain	
Superficial deficiency	Superficial palpation feels good
Internal deficiency	Deeper palpation feels good
Jitsu pain	
Superficial excess	Superficial palpation causes discomfort or pain
Internal excess	Deeper palpation causes pain

He also observed that deficient areas are not clearly demarcated (there is no clear border), whereas excess areas often have a distinct boundary.

The Tension Assessment

I can trace the roots of my personal routine for tension assessment back to my very first patient on my first nervous day of acupuncture practice back in 1987. After taking her case history, looking at her tongue and feeling her pulse, I was paralysed with indecision. I needed to buy myself more time. I started palpating her arms and legs while considering which points to use. After a few minutes of this, she looked at me with great affection in her eyes and said: "You've been doing this a long time, haven't you?"

Palpation had worked so well as a strategy for stalling that I continued to do it with every patient. As time went on, I gradually became more confident and quicker at deciding on a treatment, but by then checking muscular tension on the arms and legs had become habitual. Long before I had heard of abdominal diagnosis and the Japanese focus on stroking the channels, my palpation routine became a way to connect physically with my patients before needling. In recent years, it was a simple matter to adapt this routine for Ontake.

This tension assessment is always the first thing I do when the patient lies down, before *hara* diagnosis (abdominal diagnosis) and before taking the pulse. It is a short procedure, usually taking less than a couple of minutes. Very often, it informs the *hara* diagnosis and the final diagnosis. This kind of palpation is particularly useful

---

58   Tsuboi, K., (2008). The Application of Sanshin Technique According to The Determination of Kyojitsu, *Keiraku Chiryo – International Toyohari News*, p. 34.

when Ontake is to be used for pain relief, as it allows preliminary explorations of suitable channels to treat. For example, if using Dr Tan's mirroring system, when someone has shoulder pain, we might pay especial attention to the tops of the thighs, the corresponding treatment area (see chapter 11).

Start simply by holding the patient somewhere, perhaps the head under the occiput or the feet. As you do this, let your mind calm down and start to notice what your hands are sensing. Once you have a feeling of connection, you can start to move your hands and palpate, focusing on muscular tension, warmth, coolness and other signs of *kyo* and *jitsu*.

Tension Assessment (Supine)

1. Stroke the patient's nearest forearm two or three times on the anterior aspect and note the overall lustre.
2. Press lightly from shoulder to wrist, noting general areas of tension.
3. Pick up and squeeze from shoulder to wrist.
4. Repeat steps 2 and 3 on the leg on the same side, working from the hip to the ankle.
5. Repeat on arm and leg on the other side.
6. Put one hand on the right hip and one on the left shoulder and lean gently, stretching the two areas. Change your hands over to the right shoulder and left hip. This immediately gives you a sense of the stiffness and elasticity of the diagonal axes of the torso.
7. Check the tops of the shoulders and the sides of the neck.

Sometimes patients wear long sleeves or trousers. It is still possible to pick up much information by palpating through clothing. Even if you cannot touch the skin directly, you can still note the underlying condition of the muscles through even the heaviest of materials. Where you can, observe the skin lustre and make a note of puffiness, moisture, and temperature differences.

Tension Assessment (Prone)

The front of the body is yin, and the back of the body is yang. If the aim of treatment is to balance yin and yang, we need to treat both sides. In my experience of Japanese acupuncture, it is unusual to treat the patient on one side only. When the patient turns over, there is a second tension assessment that you can do:

1. Stroke the back, checking the lustre and look for *kyo* and *jitsu*.

2. Check the neck and sides of the waist (see *kubi koshi* in chapter 12)
3. Palpate the buttocks, thighs, and in particular, the calf muscles.

Moderating Ontake According to *Kyojitsu*

When the skin feels rough and deficient, use light tapping and rolling techniques, treating lightly at the surface. On areas that feel tighter and more excess, use stronger rolling or pressing techniques. Your perception of the depth of the reaction should inform your depth of contact with the Ontake. This feeling in the skin should also inform how much treatment to give with Ontake (see chapter 10).

How to Approach Channel Palpation

Channel palpation is a skill like any other. You have to start somewhere, usually from a place of not knowing. Once you have started, you improve through repetition and observation. If you are not used to channel palpation, you may feel unsure about its value in your practice, but the more you do the simple and quick tension assessment above, the more it will yield increasing amounts of information.

Moreover, patients like it because it grounds them. For my part, what began as a delaying tactic in my early days of practice has become an essential way for me to connect with patients when they first lie down, acclimatising them to my touch and literally feeling how they are.

We will revisit the tension assessment when looking at Ontake for the treatment of pain, and once again when looking at Hirata zones, as it is our principal guide to the selection of paired channels and zones.

Summary

Abnormal tissue findings are an important part of Japanese acupuncture and moxibustion (JAM). This includes a tactile assessment of the lustre of the skin and assessments of *kyojitsu* (deficiency-excess) in the channels.

You can start channel assessment with stroking, picking up and squeezing, and pressing—not just on the front but also on the back.

Now that we have explored ways to assess the *kyojitsu* of the channels, it's time to discuss practical strategies for treating each channel and how to apply Ontake with a metronome.

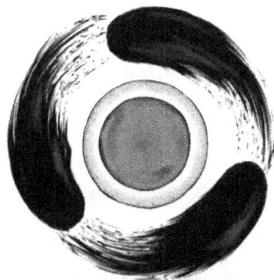

CHAPTER 6

TECHNIQUES AND FREQUENCIES

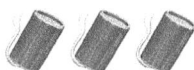

Exploring the clinical essentials of Ontake practice and covering various
techniques to apply Ontake at Manaka's meridian frequencies

Frequencies

Before we finally study techniques, it is worth considering that we are going to be
applying bamboo rhythmically, accompanied by a metronome set to a frequency of
beats per minute. The patient will hear the ticking of the metronome and feel the
sensation of the rhythmic application of heat.

Here is a simple thought experiment. Take your time, and without counting, try
tapping one arm from shoulder to wrist with your opposite hand, then go back to the
top and pick up and squeeze the muscles from shoulder to wrist.

Now repeat the process, but this time, count out loud from one to four, four
times, timing each touch or squeeze to fall on a number. What was the difference
between the two processes? Did the counting and rhythm change your perception of
applying and receiving the touch?

Before I provide an answer to this question from my perspective, now would be a good time to digress to some elementary musical theory. In the second part of the experiment above, you counted to four, four times in a row:

"One, two, three, four. One, two, three, four. One, two, three, four. One, two, three, four."

In musical terms, you just counted out four bars in 4/4 time. A bar is a measure of beats. Each group of four beats is called a bar, or measure. In the example above, there are four beats in every bar. After the fourth beat, you start counting from one again. So, when you counted to four, four times, you were counting four bars. At least since the 1960s, most songs that you have heard, especially if you like dance music, have been in 4/4 time. This time signature of four beats to one bar is embedded deep within Western popular culture.

What's more, popular songs unfold in very ordered sequences of bars. For example, an opening theme might repeat for four bars, after which a second instrument joins in. Another four bars later, the singer starts. This process is subliminal and enables skilled songwriters to fulfil or frustrate our expectations of what is coming next. As one of the aims of applying Ontake is to help your patient relax, one of the ways that you can achieve this is to make the sequence of strokes predictable.

The 4/4-time signature is very comfortable for both practitioner and patient. If you apply bamboo like this, counting the beats in your mind, it focuses your treatment, training you to repeat techniques in a subliminally predictable pattern. This can ease the transition between techniques for both you and your patient.

Manaka usually recommended tapping up to ten beats before changing to another area, sometimes as many as fifty, but I personally find this counter-intuitive, given my tendency to experience things in cycles. Contemporary practitioners and patients are steeped in a popular culture of "four-to-the-floor" music and therefore are trained to expect change that happens on the beat and in cycles.

When you take a break from this book, have a listen to a pop classic like "Hey Jude" by the Beatles and count the bars (if it's not in your collection, search YouTube or Spotify). Every significant change in the song comes at the end of an eight-bar cycle. These cycles are predictable and give the song its structure and enduring momentum. Listen to any song on the radio and count the bars and you'll find changes occurring in predictable cycles.*59 Thus, I recommend that, at least for your first few months of bamboo practice, you count in bars of four and apply techniques

---

*59 If, like me, you love dance music, you can also search for a super-infectious little dance classic called "Mucho Macho" by Dave Lee (make sure it's the Tiger Stripes Lithium Dub Mix). Once again, count the bars and enjoy how the song unfolds in predictable measures (https://youtu.be/ksirSIQ68FU).

in even numbers of bars. When you change technique, do so at the end of a cycle, not in the middle of one.

Double Time, Quarter Time, and Rapid Time

Until now, we have discussed applying bamboo in a simple rhythmic way. If the metronome clicks one, two, three, four—we tap one, two, three, four. This is very easy to grasp and quite simple to perform.

Some techniques, such as standing and leaning, however, need a lower but related frequency. Rather than standing the bamboo for one beat on the point, we might let it stand there for four or even eight beats. Even if the bamboo is static for eight beats and then moved in time to the metronome, this is still essentially the same frequency.

We can understand this by imagining the same note played at different octaves on a piano. The lower, middle, and upper notes all resonate together. In the same way, we can see that 120 beats per minute resonates with 60, 30, and 15 beats per minute. It also resonates with 240 or 480 beats per minute. These are all points along the same fundamental frequency continuum.

All music exploits these frequency relationships to the basic time signature, and when applying bamboo, we can exploit them, too, even without being virtuoso musicians.

In the example above, standing technique with bamboo would involve keeping the bamboo in place for eight beats or two bars before moving it to the next place. If the frequency is 120 beats per minute, we are applying the frequency four times more slowly. Slowing down feels nice, sometimes. We don't have to change the metronome from 120 beats per minute, of course. All we need to do is count to four or eight before moving the bamboo.

We can also speed up. Tapping is a technique frequently applied over a broad area, such as the upper back and shoulders. It can be useful to tap in double time. Again, there is no need to adjust the metronome, only the way you count and tap. Instead of tapping, "One, two, three, four; one, two, three, four," you tap:

"One and two and three and four, and one and two and three and four and... ".

Tapping in this way covers a broader area more quickly, and once again, a change of rhythm is a change of energy.

Finally, there is the highest frequency variation. For this, you need to practise a little. This is a rapid oscillation of the hand from side to side, four times faster than the base frequency. Visually this looks something like this:

$$1^{234}, 2^{234}, 3^{234}, 4^{234}, 1^{234}, 2^{234}, 3^{234}, 4^{234}$$

Performed on a drum, this would be a drumroll. When applied to the skin, it generates a warm, penetrating vibration.

Nine and Six (*Jiu Liu*)

There is one final question to consider about rhythm. Within acupuncture traditions, there are many references to even numbers being yin and odd numbers being yang. Here's how French author and TCM practitioner Bernard Auteroche described this:

> This technique is based on the theory of the *I Ching*, and associates Yin with even numbers, and Yang with odd numbers. Broadly speaking, the odd number 9, which is Yang, is used to reinforce, and the even number 6, which is Yin, is used to reduce.
>
> To reinforce, the needle should be thrust in forcefully and lifted gently 9 times… repeated in multiples of 9.
>
> To reduce, the needle should be thrust in gently and withdrawn strongly 6 times, [and] repeated in multiples of 6.[60]

Moreover, when you read moxibustion prescriptions, the number of cones recommended is usually odd. Sung Baek, a moxibustion specialist and author of an influential book on moxibustion, recommends three to seven cones on one point, or three to nine cones daily, increasing over time to eleven daily.[61]

If odd numbers are good for needle techniques and cone numbers, should we consider them for time signatures for bamboo? I have experimented with various yin and yang time signatures, namely three, five, six and seven beats per bar. All of them work, but I cannot say whether they work better or worse than four beats per bar. They are, however, slightly harder to apply, and at a subliminal level, they are stranger to receive than "four-to-the-floor" tapping. However, there have been occasions where a stubborn tight area that did not respond to 4/4 techniques yielded to a 7/4 routine. Whether this was because of the change of time signature or the reapplication of bamboo a second time, I cannot say.

---

60   Auteroche, B. (1992). *Acupuncture and Moxibustion: A Guide to Clinical Practice*. Edinburgh: Churchill Livingstone, p. 47.

61   Baek, S. (1990). *Classical Moxibustion Skills in Contemporary Clinical Practice*. Boulder, CO: Blue Poppy Press, p. 3.

This question of yin and yang time signatures is a much easier to raise than to answer, especially for a single mad scientist in one clinic room in Malaysia. It is a much better question for group study and research. The numbers of Ontake practitioners worldwide are growing, and using online communities on Facebook or Sayoshi.com (an online directory for practitioners of JAM), we could devise a study protocol to explore this issue.

Hands On

You have palpated the patient, and you have an idea that they are kind of tight *there* and sort of weak *here*. Your bamboo is loaded and lit. This is all you need to get started.

It is useful to think of Ontake as a highly versatile, heated, pressing tool. Its different parts—the base, the lip, or the sides—can be applied to the skin. Different motions and vectors can be imparted to the bamboo, such as vertical tapping, rocking from side to side, oblique pressing, and horizontal rolling. But the secret to applying bamboo is the supplementing strokes to *kyo* areas and the draining strokes to *jitsu* areas.

Holding the Bamboo

There are no rules for where to hold the bamboo. This varies depending on which technique you are using and how hot it is. What you should always do, however, is keep your shoulder, elbow, and wrist loose and your grip on the bamboo relaxed. Some of the strokes below derive from Tui Na and Shiatsu, and both these therapies emphasise fluidity of movement and centred relaxation from the therapist. The tighter you hold the bamboo, the less relaxing it feels.

We have talked about acupuncture as a doorbell, sending a signal from the outside of the body to the inside. We have all heard visitors express their mood through the way they have rung the doorbell in our own homes. It is easy to convey humour, expectation, or irritation by ringing the doorbell in a certain way. *Bamboo communicates your level of tension to the patient.* Stay relaxed, and your touch communicates relaxation. Easier said than done.

Role of the Right Hand

Hold the bamboo in your dominant hand. Your grip should be gentle and relaxed. Keep your shoulder and elbow loose and your wrist supple. Your movements should be fluid and rhythmic. If the bamboo feels too hot to hold, hold it higher up where it is cooler. In that case, you should keep the bamboo moving quite fast so that the contact time with the skin is shorter. This is particularly important when treating the face and neck.

Role of the Left Hand

The bamboo is always in motion, moving along the area to be treated. Use your left hand as a sensor. It should always be scouting ahead of the bamboo, feeling out the *kyojitsu* along the way, so that you can adjust your technique with your right hand. Furthermore, you should use your left hand to check on changes in the wake of the bamboo. Monitor the skin for improvements in lustre and temperature, and the deeper tissues for changes in hardness. The left hand, too, can move in time to the metronome.

As you get more practised, you may notice changes in muscle tone through the bamboo as you apply it. This uses the same proprioceptive mechanisms that enable you to feel a stone at the tip of your shovel when gardening.

Practical Ontake Techniques

Cold Practice

The directions below describe how to apply lighted bamboo on a patient. For learning and practice, however, it is much better to start with an unlit bamboo and a fluffy cushion. In training sessions, we call this cold practice. Start unaccompanied, then when you feel confident, turn on the metronome and repeat the technique to one of the lower frequencies. Some of these techniques can be found on YouTube, where you can see the techniques demonstrated on a cushion. The link and timecodes for each technique are given as footnotes below, but if the link no longer works at the time of reading, simply search YouTube for The Ontake Channel and see what comes up.

Tapping

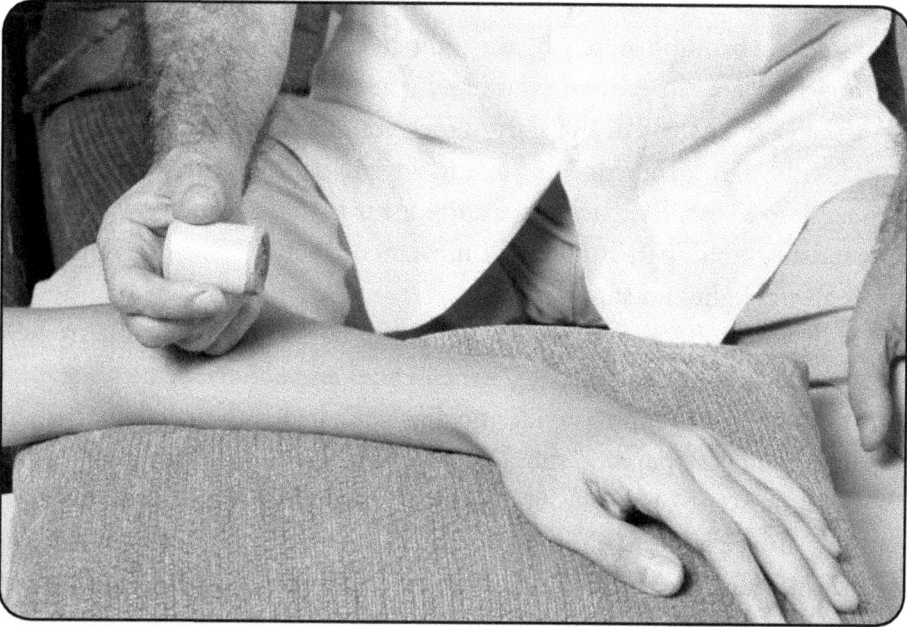

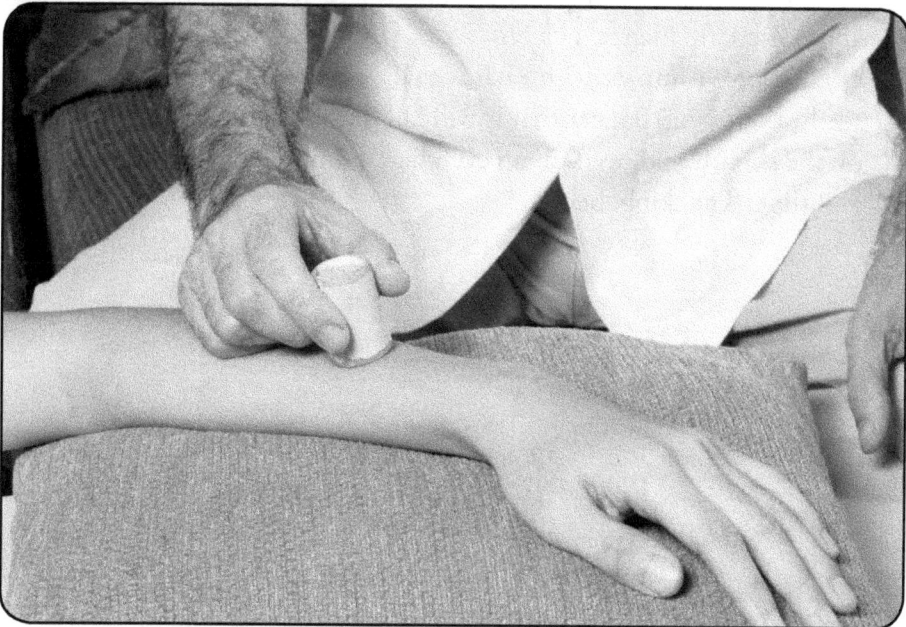

A light and supple movement: the edge of your hand acts as a fulcrum.

There are two variations of this. One emphasises the rhythmic delivery of heat to the skin, and the second emulates gentle percussion with the wooden hammer.

1. Hold the bamboo loosely by the unlit end between thumb, index, and third fingers. Place the edge of your hand (the hypothenar eminence) just below the area to be treated, and start to rock your hand so that the bamboo lightly taps the skin. The edge of your hand will act as a fulcrum, allowing the bamboo to oscillate backwards and forwards, and up and down. This is very similar to rolling in Tui Na. The movement should come from the wrist and is always light and supple.[62]

2. Shift your grip slightly further down the bamboo so that you are holding it securely in the middle. With the lighted end about one centimetre above the skin, start tapping while moving your hand up and down in parallel lines. Only the bamboo should contact the skin, not your wrist. This action is reminiscent of the motion used when shaking a salt cellar over a nice unhealthy plate of fish and chips. This technique is useful for tapping on broad areas, such as the upper back and shoulders. It is similar to tapotement in Swedish massage.

   For loose, deficient areas, tap the heated end lightly on the skin at the appropriate frequency. For *jitsu* areas, tap more percussively so that there is a sensation of impact with each tap. If you have compressed the plug correctly, there is no danger that it will fall out or that loose particles will drop on the skin. If you need to tap even harder, more percussively, see knocking and super-knocking, below.

---

62   Ontake Warm Bamboo Part 1 (2.57). YouTube. https://youtu.be/uU-hetc2Hi0

Touching and Closing

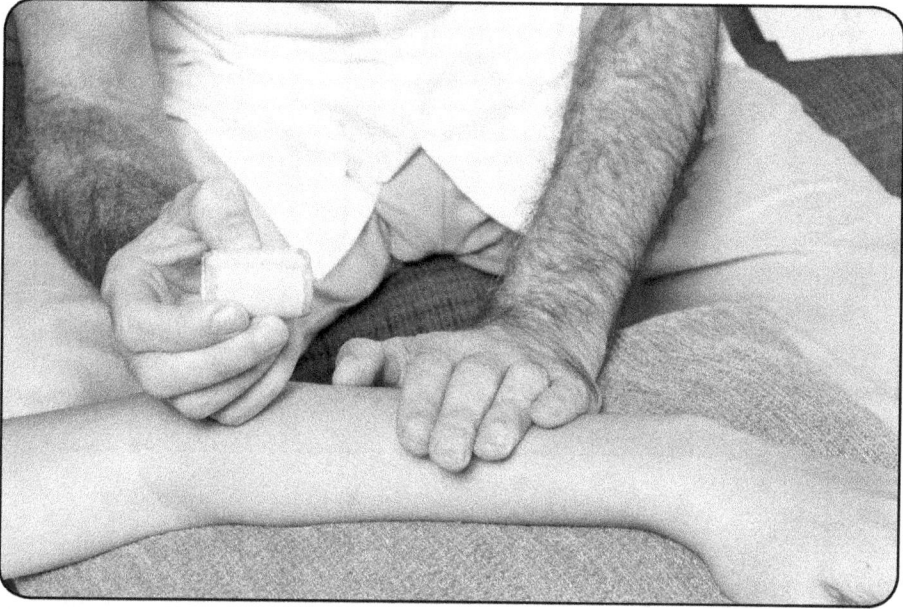

Pivot the bamboo downwards, as in tapping.

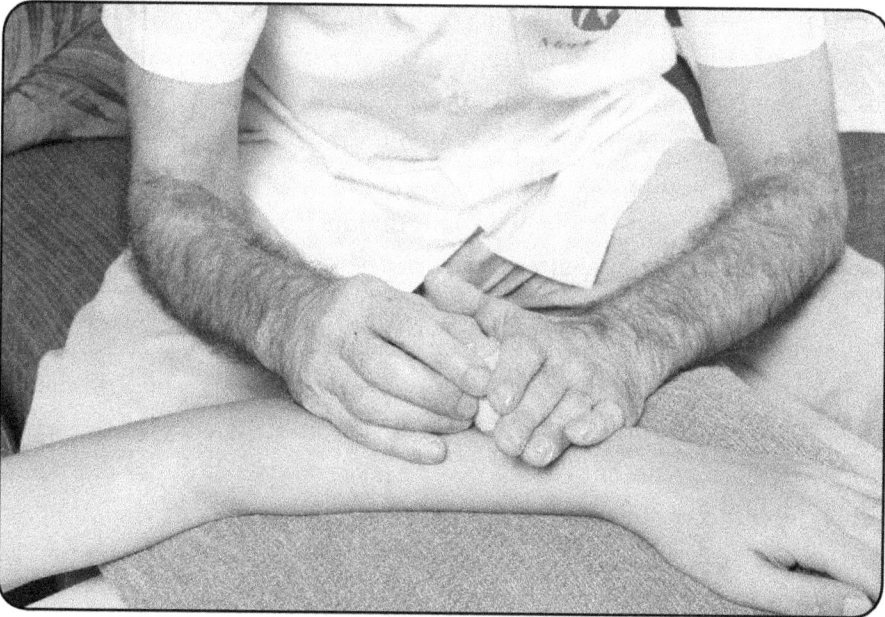

Slide your left index finger down the side of the bamboo, in time to the beat, palm flat.

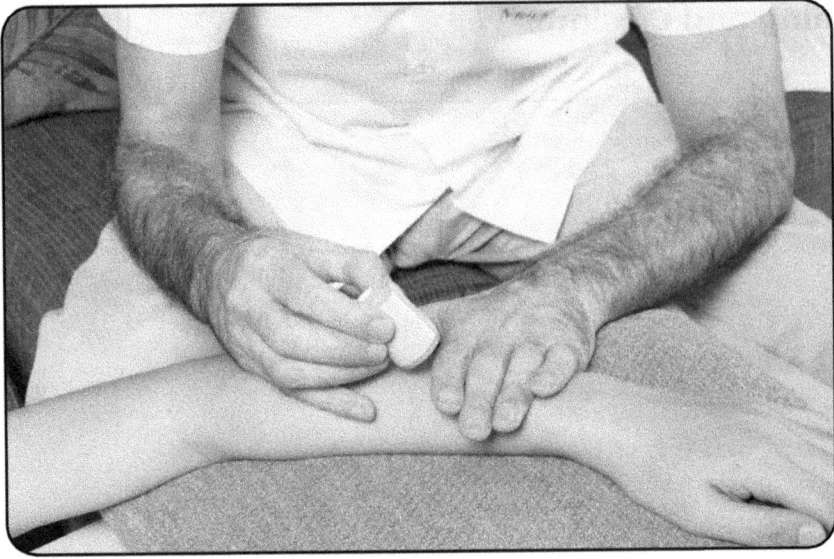

Your left hand seals in the heat.

The movement with the right hand is similar to that of step 1 of tapping, above. Hold the bamboo in your right hand, then place and remove it softly and rhythmically on the skin. As you remove it, slide your left index finger down the side of the bamboo, keeping your palm flat, facing downwards, with your fingers together. Press your left hand softly on the skin. Move the bamboo slightly to the right and repeat. Your left hand "closes" the area treated by the bamboo and pushes or seals the heat in further. Keep moving to the right, sealing in the heat. If you do several passes over the same area, you can monitor the skin temperature changes with your left hand as you press down.

This is a very soft and supplementing technique for *kyo* areas, equivalent to an acupuncturist closing the hole after removing the needle or a very gentle (and safe) version of press moxa with a moxa stick.

This technique is one of the most useful techniques to master and feels pleasant both to give and receive. It is a hard technique to visualise just by reading; even in class, some students find the coordination of left and right hands the hardest to grasp. One familiar precedent from daily life is the simple action of grating cheese. When touching and closing in time to a metronome, the left hand should be tapping the skin on the beat, using the same kind of coordination as when grating a piece of cheese with an upright grater. The left hand is like the cheese, and the bamboo is the grater. The left hand follows the metronome and connects with the skin on the downbeat; the right hand pulls the bamboo away and replaces it on the offbeat.[63]

---

63   Ontake Warm Bamboo Part 1 (3.20). YouTube. https://youtu.be/uU-hetc2Hi0

Rolling

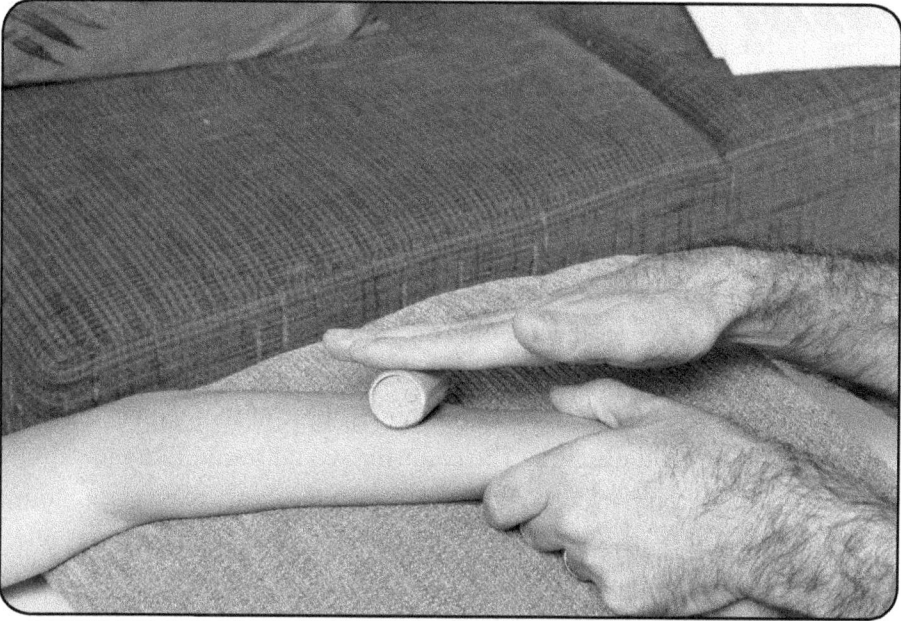

Rolling lightly.

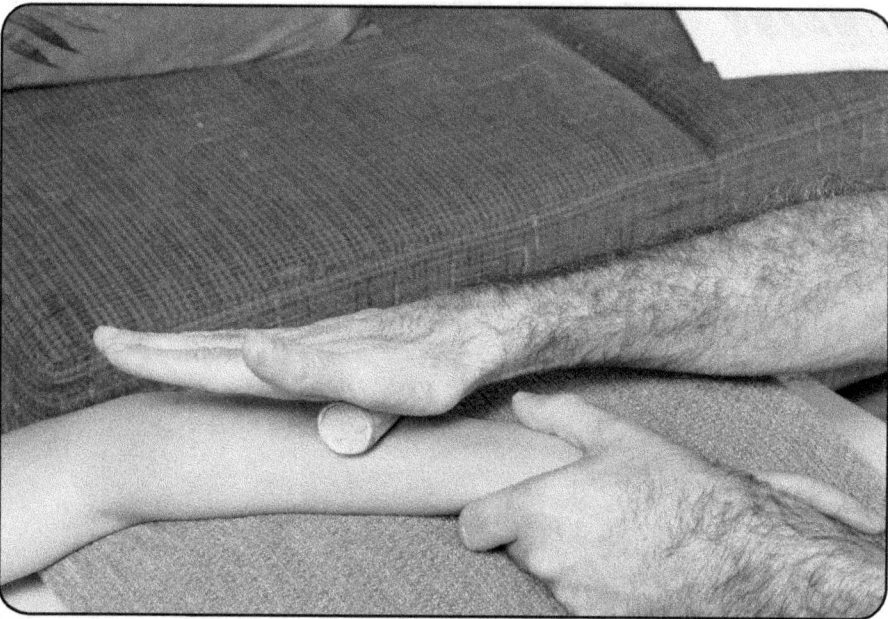

Rolling more deeply.

Rolling is one of the most pleasant and effective strokes to receive with bamboo and is immediately suggested by its cylindrical shape. Roll the bamboo rhythmically on the skin with the palmar surface of your right hand. You can vary the pressure, rolling lightly for areas of cool or loose skin and more firmly for muscle tension deeper inside. For lighter pressure, keep the bamboo more under your fingers. For stronger pressure, keep it more under your palm. Thus, rolling can be used for *ho* and *sha,* depending on how hard you apply it.[64]

Sometimes you end up "rolling yourself into a corner". For example, you may roll all the way down the back and find yourself at the sacrum with nowhere to go. You can use your little finger and thumb to pick up and move the bamboo to another area while still keeping in rhythm. Practise this on your thigh. When you reach the knee, pick up the bamboo, and in time to the beat, bring it back to the top of your thigh.

You can do the pick-up or recovery on the last beat of the bar, rolling for seven beats and picking up on the eighth. The counting would sound like this:

One, two, three, four, five, six, seven-and-pick-up, one, two, three, four, five, six, seven-and-pick-up, one, two, three, four, five, six, seven-and-pick-up, one, two, three, four, five, six, seven-and-pick-up.

Standing

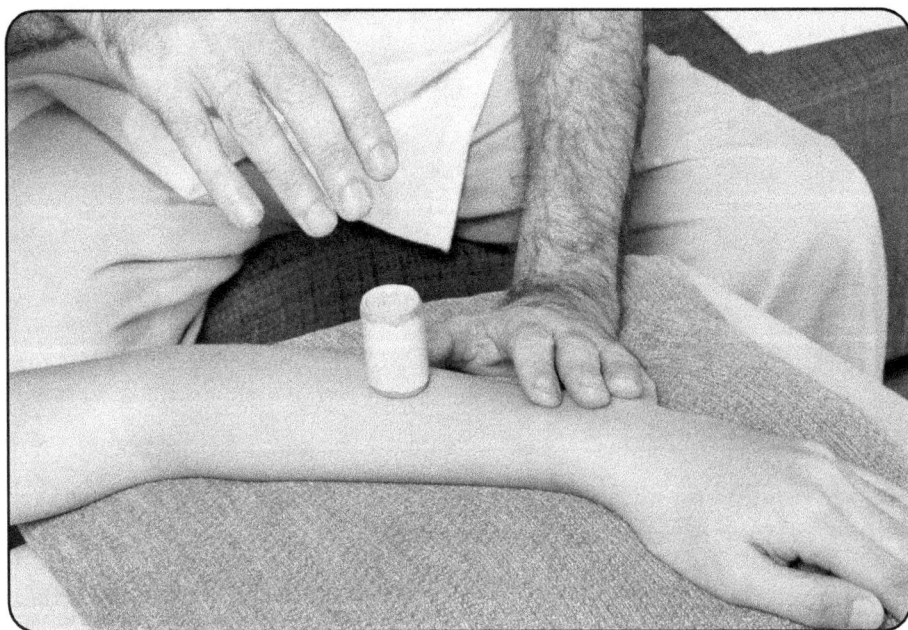

A little like playing chess, pick up and move the piece.

---

64   Ontake Warm Bamboo Part 1 (3.55). YouTube. https://youtu.be/uU-hetc2Hi0

Place the bamboo vertically on a specific point with the heated end facing down. Leave for four or eight beats and then move it to the next place. This supplementing technique feels very comfortable on areas like the lower Du Mai points or the sacrum. If treating a single point, such as ST 36, stand for four beats and remove for four beats. This technique introduces the concept that we explored earlier—namely, that the frequency can be effective even when the bamboo moves at a slower rate than the metronome. Here we are keeping to the frequency but moving only after one or two bars. It feels a bit like moving a chess piece.[65]

Rocking

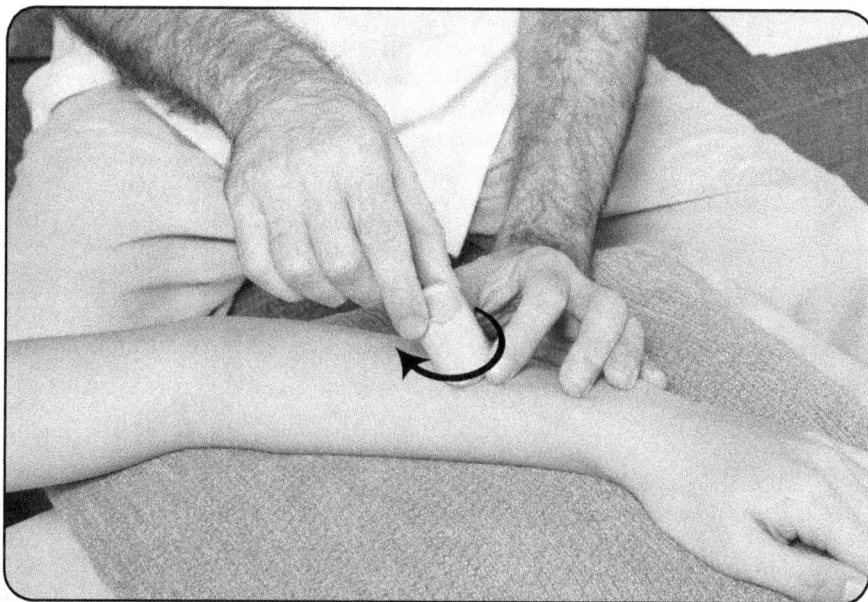

Rotate the bamboo on the skin as if you were stirring a cup of tea.

Rocking is a more dynamic form of treating one point than standing. Hold the base of the bamboo on the point, between the thumb and index finger of your left hand (*oshide*). With the thumb and index finger of your right hand (*sashide*) holding the top of the bamboo, make a stirring motion, like stirring a cup of tea, so that the bamboo is rocking rhythmically over the point. Rock for one to four bars, taking care not to overheat the point.[66]

---

65   Ontake Warm Bamboo Part 1 (4.28). YouTube. https://youtu.be/uU-hetc2Hi0
66   Ontake Warm Bamboo Part 1 (4.57). YouTube. https://youtu.be/uU-hetc2Hi0

Pressing

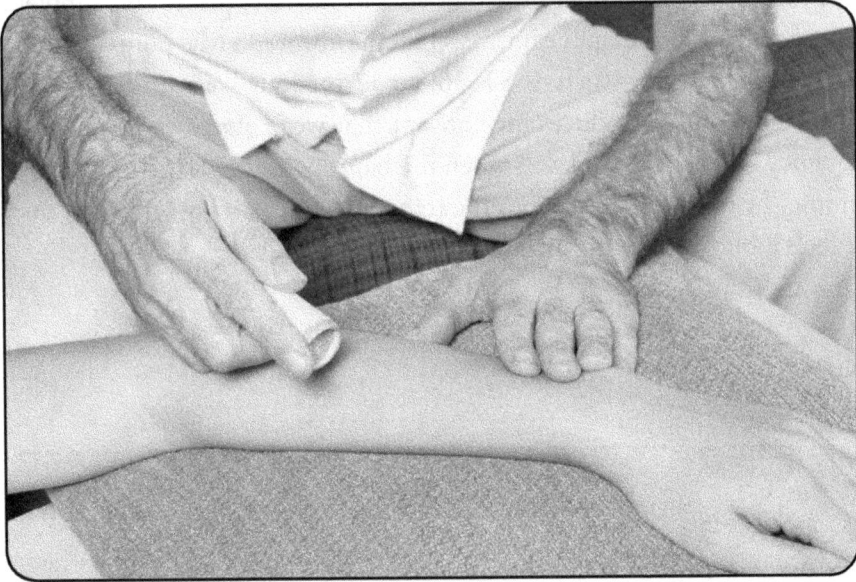

Hold the bamboo between the thumb and third finger, with
your index finger extended across the long axis.

Pressing is a wonderful exploratory technique that gives you much information about the general tone of an area, even as you start to treat it. There is also a variation that can be used in a focused way around joints and muscle insertions.

1. With your palm facing up, place the bamboo flat onto your third finger, moving your second and fourth fingers up a little to create a trough where it can nest. Grip the side of the bamboo with your thumb and rotate your palm so that you can place the side of the bamboo on the area to be treated. Next press the warm side of the bamboo against the muscle in a fluid, repetitive motion. This can be used on either side of the spine on the bladder channel or on the upper arm and shoulder.

2. Hold the bamboo between the thumb and third finger, with your index finger extended across the long axis. With the bamboo angled at roughly forty-five degrees, press down rhythmically into tight areas with the warm lip. This technique is useful for *jitsu* areas—for example, the medial border of the scapula. It helps to give a slight twist to the bamboo as you press down and then release.[67]

67　　Ontake Warm Bamboo Part 1 (5.32). YouTube. https://youtu.be/uU-hetc2Hi0

Knocking

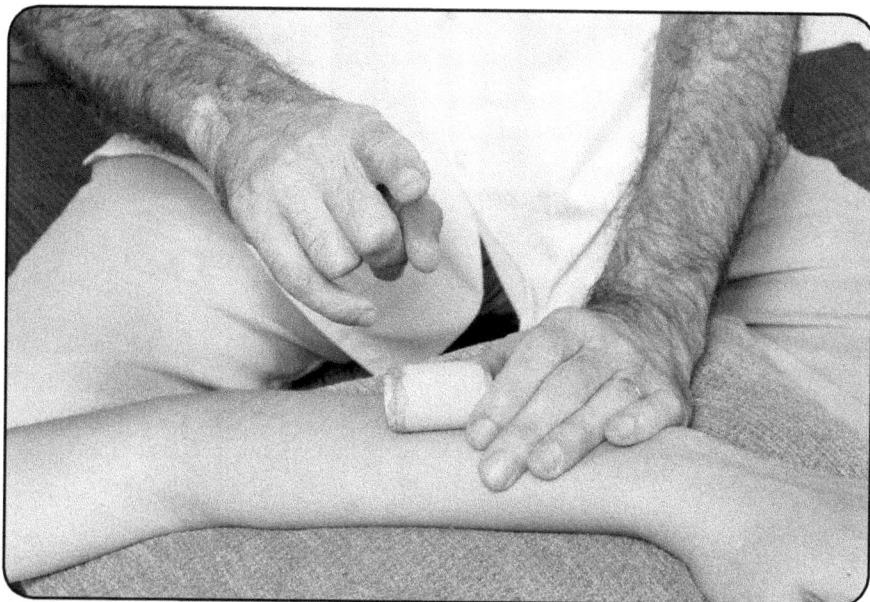

With the bamboo on its side, tap it firmly with one or two fingers.

Place the hot bamboo on its side on the area to treat, and then tap it firmly with one or two fingers. This safely combines percussive elements of Manaka's wooden needle treatment with the application of heat. Pick up the bamboo after one or two bars and move it to the next point. To increase the percussive element, you can use your knuckle to knock the bamboo, exactly like knocking on someone's door. This kind of knocking can be used on tight and painful points, such as on the abdomen or in between the thoracic vertebrae. Bear in mind that the longer you leave the bamboo in one place, the hotter it feels, so don't forget to keep the bamboo in motion every one or two bars.[68]

68   Ontake Warm Bamboo Part 1 (1.54). YouTube. https://youtu.be/uU-hetc2Hi0

Super-knocking

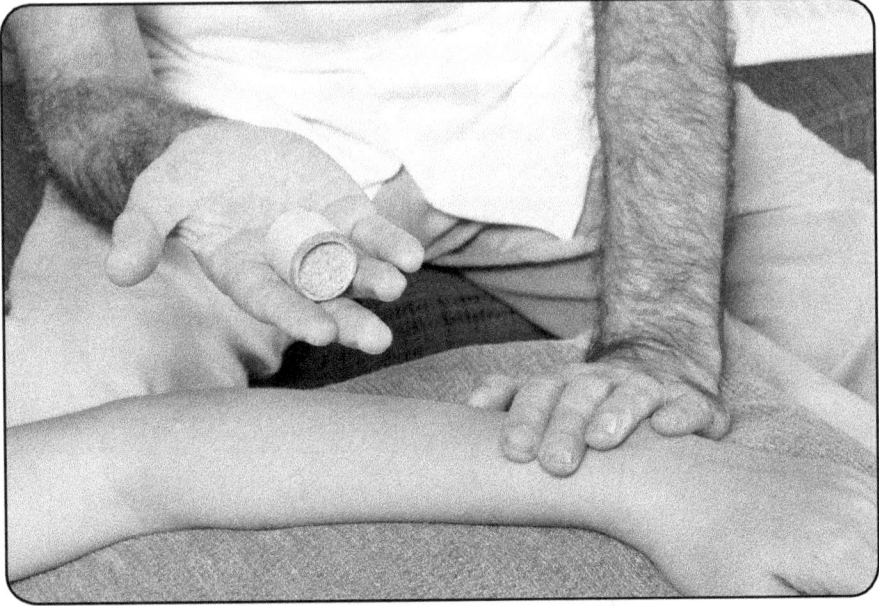

Nest the bamboo in the trough between your second and
fourth fingers, then turn your hand over.

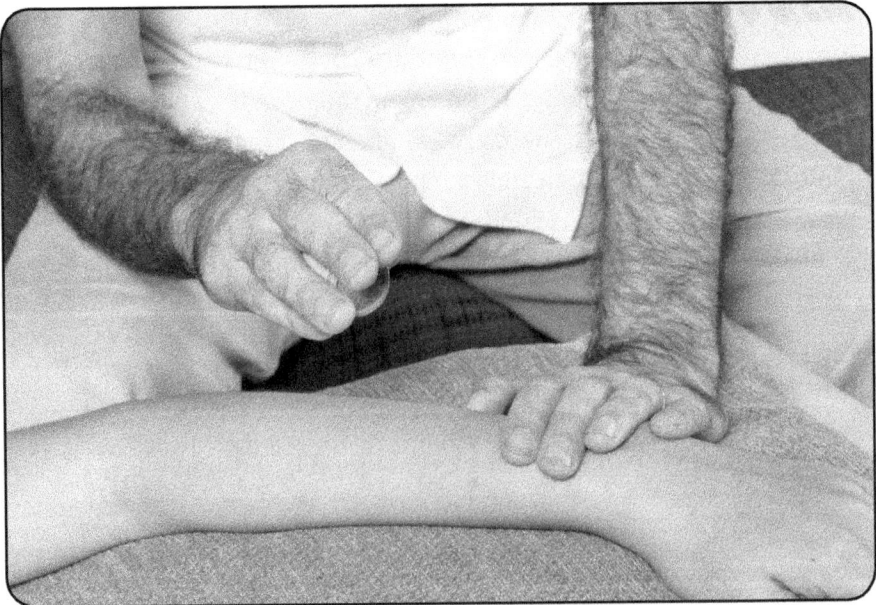

Tap lightly but forcefully with the side of the bamboo.

After a few minutes of use, the entire length of the bamboo, not just the smouldering end, becomes warm. A more dynamic variation of knocking is to bounce or "strike" the side of the bamboo with some force, against the skin. Hold the bamboo as you would for pressing, longitudinally in the trough created by your middle three fingers and strike the muscles lightly but forcefully, so that you create a percussive wave in the soft tissue.

This again combines percussive elements of Manaka's wooden needle treatment with the rhythmic application of heat and is excellent for softening muscular or *jitsu* areas of soft tissue, such as the buttocks, thigh, calf, or deltoids. It feels very relaxing. This technique is not suitable for bony areas.[69]

Leaning

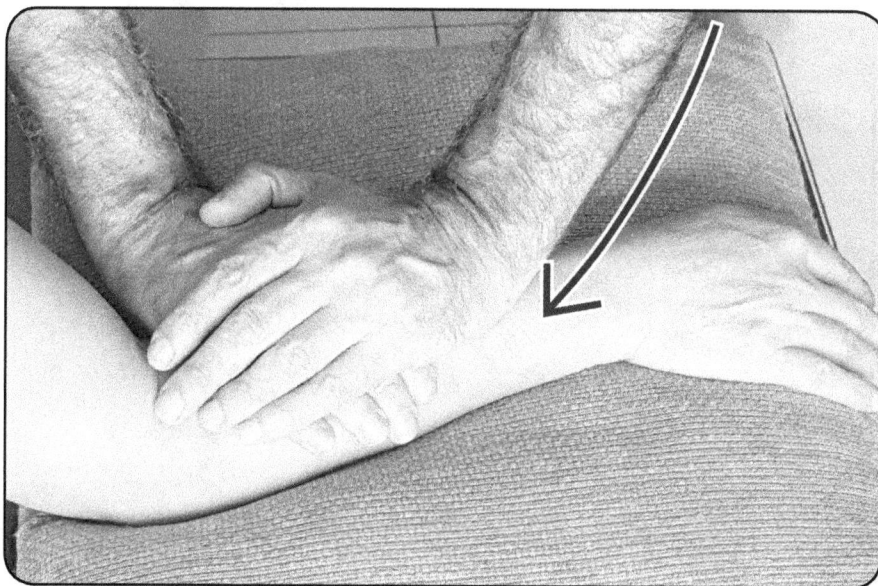

Lean your weight through your top hand into your bottom hand and into the bamboo.

This technique comes directly from Shiatsu. In Shiatsu, it is important to apply pressure with the weight of your body and not by using the muscular strength of your arms. In this way, your muscles stay relaxed and open and are therefore able to move qi. Using our doorbell analogy, we can take "moving qi" to mean that we send a signal of relaxation, through our own relaxed state, that is received by the patient's body.

---

69   Ontake Warm Bamboo Part 1 (2.17). YouTube. https://youtu.be/uU-hetc2Hi0

Lay the bamboo flat on the skin and cover it with the palm of your left hand. Now cover your left hand with your right. Lean your body weight down into your right hand, keeping both arms relaxed so that the bamboo is pressed down into the deeper layers. Count four or eight beats and then move the bamboo to the next point, taking care not to overheat the skin. This technique is useful for indurations on the lower lumbar area, abdomen, and the back of the legs and should be followed immediately by rolling to further move the blood. You can reverse this if you are left-handed. The principle is to lean your weight with the top hand into the bottom hand and down into the bamboo.[70]

Vibrating

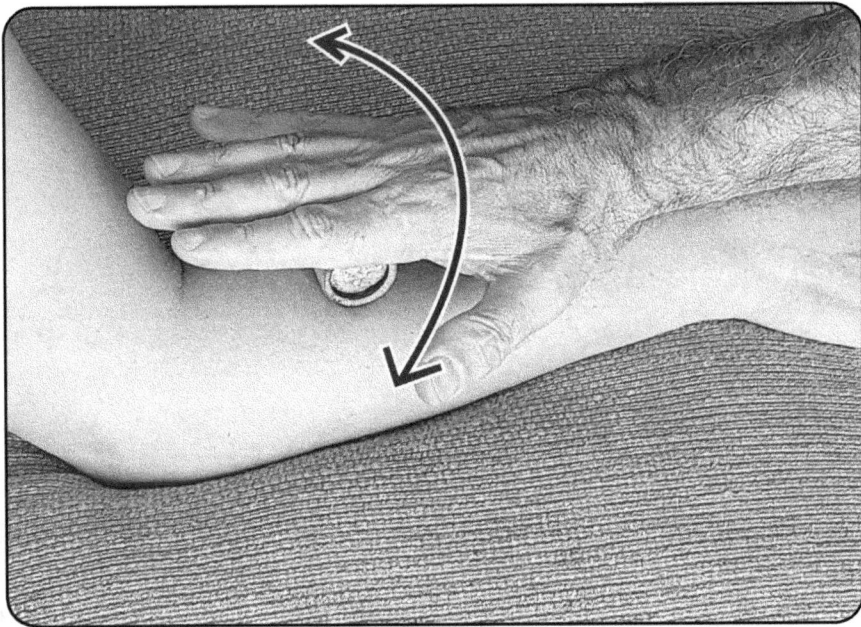

Vibrate your palm rapidly from side to side, with minimal amplitude.

These final three techniques require mastering the hardest of the frequency variations discussed above: the rapid oscillation of the hand, four times faster than the base frequency. It is not as hard as it sounds and has such impressive effects it is well worth taking time to practise. If you are already a musician, you will get it right away.

---

70   Ontake Warm Bamboo Part 1 (6.22). YouTube. https://youtu.be/uU-hetc2Hi0

Place the bamboo flat on its side on the point to be treated, and cover it with your palm. Now vibrate your palm rapidly from side to side, with minimal amplitude, in time to the beat but four times faster. This produces a pleasing, spreading sensation of warmth at the point and can be very useful to deploy on stiff, tight areas or meeting points with unique properties, such as DU 14. Once again, it is worth emphasising that you need to keep your movements light, relaxed, and subtle. This is not the vibration of a mechanical digger smashing up a road; it is the airy vibration of a dragonfly's wings over a pond.[71]

Bouncing

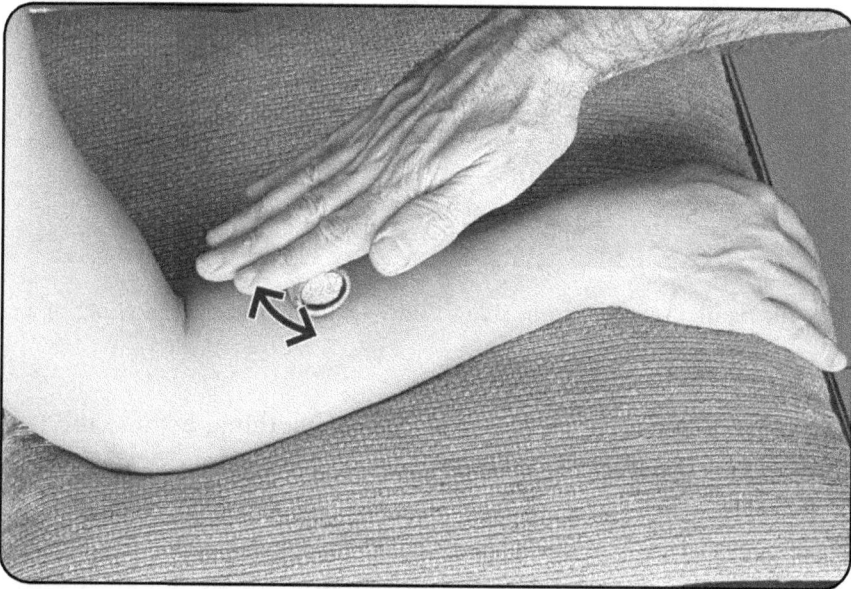

Oscillate your fingers up and down rapidly, with minimal amplitude.

This technique is only suitable for fleshy areas and cannot be used comfortably on joints or bony areas. As with vibrating, place the bamboo on the point to be treated, and cover it with your fingers, as in light rolling. This time, instead of vibrating your hand from side to side, oscillate your fingers with an up-and-down movement with minimal amplitude, allowing the bamboo to bounce rapidly on the soft tissue. Once again, this produces a spreading sensation of warmth and relaxation and can be used to release tightness on fleshy areas, such as the calf, deltoid, or waist.

---

71   Ontake Warm Bamboo Part 1 (6.59). YouTube. https://youtu.be/uU-hetc2Hi0

Rubbing

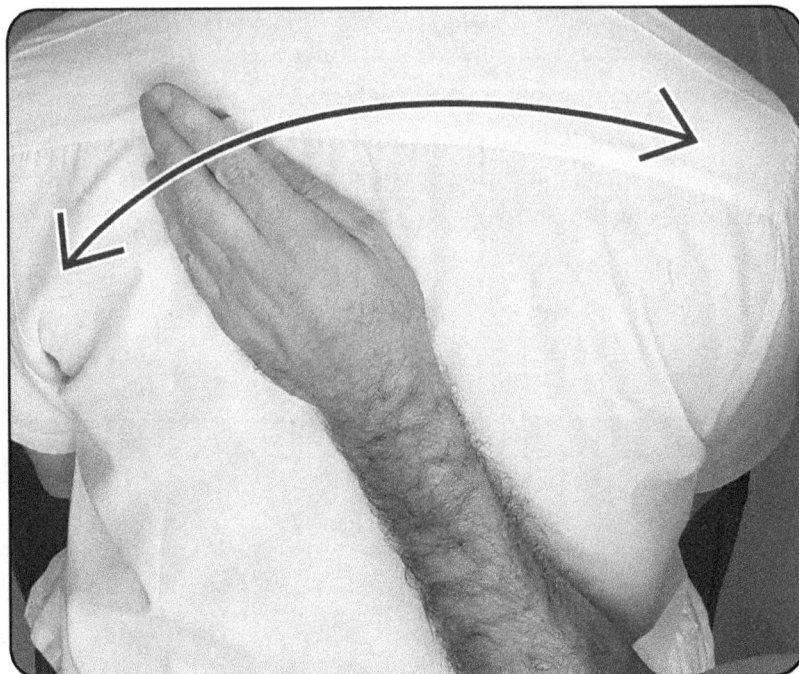

Sweep the bamboo rapidly from side to side—like the windscreen wiper of a car.

This last technique is excellent to use through clothing, because the fabric of a shirt or trouser leg enables virtually frictionless gliding over a broad area. Place the bamboo flat on the area to be treated, and grasp it loosely with your thumb, index and third fingers. This time, sweep the bamboo rapidly from side to side, covering a wide arc with each sweep—like the windscreen wiper of a car, but much faster. Hold the bamboo so lightly that it skates across the skin or fabric. Once again, this rapid oscillatory movement can produce surprising results. Patients love it. This technique is particularly useful on the upper or lower back.

Techniques Divided by Function

As we have seen, the objective of traditional acupuncture in general is to regulate the flow of qi and blood by balancing *kyo* and *jitsu* in the channels. Where the skin and muscles feel weak and deficient, we apply milder bamboo techniques to supplement deficiency. Where the skin and tissues feel tight and with excess, we apply more moving or draining techniques to break up the stagnation and move qi and blood.

MOXA IN MOTION   83

Some techniques are purely supplementing, and others are purely draining. Other techniques—rolling, for example—can be used both to supplement and to drain by moderating the intensity of application.

Below is a table showing the techniques and their general functions.

Table 7 Technique Modalities

Technique	*Ho* (Supplementing)	*Sha* (Draining)
Tapping	•	•
Touching and closing	•	
Rolling	•	•
Standing	•	
Rocking	•	
Pressing	•	•
Knocking		•
Super-knocking		•
Leaning		•
Vibrating	•	•
Bouncing		•
Rubbing	•	•

One final point to make about the techniques above is that only two of them, standing and rocking, are aimed at treating acupuncture points. Every other technique is designed to treat broad areas or lines along the flow of a channel. Thus, the thinking behind bamboo is different than that of conventional moxibustion and acupuncture, focusing on zones rather than points. This becomes especially relevant when considering the systemic and distal effects of warming channels and zones when using holographic systems, such as those developed by Dr Richard Tan or Kurakichi Hirata.

Metronomes

This chapter should close with a discussion of metronomes. In Manaka's day, dedicated metronomes were only one electronic step up from the old clockwork ones. These days, your smartphone can support a wide selection of metronome apps, sophisticated and accurate enough to satisfy professional musicians.

One of my patients, a musician in the Malaysian Philharmonic Orchestra, observed that my free metronome app was not keeping accurate time. She recommended a more advanced paid app used by professionals (see appendix for resources). This more sophisticated kind of metronome, apart from being accurate, can be programmed to produce natural-sounding clicks that are easy on the ear. Most importantly, for practitioners unfamiliar with Manaka's frequencies, you can create a playlist of your favourite songs, or in our case, frequencies. This means that rather than manually scrolling from say, 152 to 104 beats per minute, you can easily switch from one of the eight frequencies to another.

Electronic metronomes built into your phone have many advantages, but they also have some drawbacks that can compromise your treatment, not least of which are notifications from other apps that may distract you during your treatment. For this reason, when using my phone in clinic, I switch it to airplane mode. Other considerations about metronomes are discussed below.

Click Sounds

Most metronomes allow you to select the type of sound. These vary from robotic electronic beeps to maraca sounds to woodblock sounds. I strongly recommend a natural sound. Robotic beeps are reminiscent of alarm clocks and Casio keyboards and watches, whereas wood blocks are more natural and, arguably, may remind us of our tribal origins.

Click Volume

Your phone speaker needs to be loud enough for you to hear above the sound of you applying the treatment. If applying wooden hammer and needle, you may need to turn the volume up slightly; otherwise, the sound of the hammer hitting the needle drowns out the sound of the metronome, and you may begin to lose time.

As applying Ontake is almost silent, your metronome does not need to be loud. If you set the volume high—and the internal speaker of an iPad can certainly go very loud—it can start to feel oppressive, the opposite of what you intend.

Click Emphasis

Metronome apps come with a facility to emphasise the first beat of the bar. Sometimes there is a default setting to create an accent on one beat:

"*One*, two, three, four. *One*, two, three, four."

Apps achieve this by changing the sound on that beat—for example, by making it higher-pitched and louder. Once again, this works against the subliminal relaxation of the therapy. In 4/4 time, the louder click becomes too predictable and mechanical, limiting the fluidity of your strokes. In other time signatures, such as 7/4 or 5/4, the louder click does the opposite, emphasising the unpredictability of the sequence. Moreover, and especially at higher volumes, that super-regular digital accent can start to sound too mechanical—even irritating—and can overpower the gentle aims of treatment.

In all cases, I recommend that there should be no emphasis on any beat. The sound of your metronome should be intentionally anodyne.

Any of these three pitfalls can end up sabotaging your treatment. The way to avoid them is to remember these three simple rules:

- Choose a natural sound.
- Keep the volume low.
- Set the app to play with no accent.

Summary

Communication with your patient is a two-way street. You can detect muscle tension through the tension assessment or with your left hand, but you can communicate your own tension through the way you hold the bamboo. Always try to keep your shoulders, arms, and wrist open and loose.

There are many techniques and variations that you can employ. Use lighter techniques for *kyo* areas and firmer techniques for *jitsu* areas. For the most part, use "four-to-the-floor" time signatures that feel predictable and comforting.

Remember to keep your phone sounds natural, quiet, and without emphasis.

The best way to put all this together is to grab a colleague or family member and treat them from top to bottom with bamboo. In chapter 8 we learn how to do exactly that: whole body routines that integrate everything we have covered so far. But first, let's have a think about the mechanisms of Ontake and what it might actually be doing.

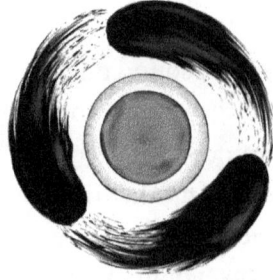

CHAPTER 7

ACTIONS, CONTRAINDICATIONS, AND APPLICATIONS

Exploring the possible mechanisms of Ontake treatment, listing its functions in TEAM thinking. Examining the standard contraindications for moxibustion to extrapolate what may be the contraindications for Ontake.

The Many Mechanisms of Ontake

Before we launch into a discussion of Ontake's practical applications, now would be a good time to conjecture briefly on its actions and contraindications. Ontake has been around for a relatively short time, and little has been written about it in Japanese, let alone in English. We therefore have to figure out for ourselves what it does and what contraindications might be appropriate.

Manaka and his colleague Kazuko Itaya suggested that the action of the wooden hammer and needle was similar to that of a shallowly inserted needle.[72] When the

---

72   Manaka, Y., Itaya, K., & Birch, S. (1995). *Chasing the Dragon's Tail: The Theory and Practice of Acupuncture in the Work of Yoshio Manaka.* Brookline: Paradigm Publications.

wooden needle is tapped more vigorously, so that the vibrations are felt as a radiating sensation, the effects resemble those of deeper needling.

As you will see when you start to use bamboo, it can rapidly relieve chronic stagnation, tightness and pain in the soft tissue. Those tight upper shoulders that take so much painful pressing and rubbing with oil-based massages simply melt in seconds when treated with bamboo. It may be, therefore, that the actions of bamboo, combined with the percussive effects of the wooden hammer with the radiant and heat-conductive effects of moxibustion, work at the deeper level of blood.

Sung Baek, a moxibustion specialist and author of an influential book on moxibustion, differentiates the effects of needling, moxibustion, and bloodletting on the body.[73] Needling accesses the pre-existing energy of the body, and moxibustion adds energy to the body. Bloodletting physically drains energy out of the body. Thus, we have three modalities to regulate qi and blood, all with very different kinds of effects.

The effects of bamboo appear to straddle the first two of these modalities. It works on the qi level and the blood level, and much of its effects on these levels come from the techniques that resemble its predecessor, Manaka's wooden needle with the meridian frequencies (see chapter 4). However, bamboo also uses heat from moxa and can therefore be considered useful for supplementing and adding energy into the system. Moreover, when the heat is combined with more vigorous strokes such as leaning and deep rolling (see chapter 5), it has a powerful effect on moving the blood.

Ontake communicates with the body on all sorts of levels. Before you approach the patient, they hear the sound of the metronome and smell the moxa smoke. Particularly if this is a repeat treatment, these sounds and smells serve as anchors that immediately relax the patient, reminding them of previous relaxed Ontake states. These anchors were vividly described by a patient of mine whose baby had colic. For the first few days, he would cry when he was in pain, but he got immediate relief when she lit the Ontake and warmed his tummy. After a few days, as soon as he heard the distinctive clicking of the lighter and the hissing of the gas as the Ontake was lit, his tummy would relax, and he would stop crying before she even brought the Ontake close.

Next, there are mechanical effects from rolling and pressing (see chapter 6), similar to physical therapy strokes such as effleurage, petrissage, and friction, which all improve blood circulation in the Western physiological sense. With some of the more percussive techniques, there is an effect similar to techniques used in chiropractic, such as Activator Therapy—a method that uses a sprung hammer to tap joints and soft tissues.

---

73   Baek, S. (1990). *Classical Moxibustion Skills in Contemporary Clinical Practice*. Boulder, CO: Blue Poppy Press.

Once you contact the skin with the lit Ontake, there may also be pharmacological effects with the absorption of the biochemical products of moxibustion into the skin. Certainly, the skin can smell smoky after treatment. In TCM, the smoke from moxa is thought to have healing properties of its own, which has led to techniques, such as *ai xun jiu*, that consciously attempt to fumigate the skin or joints.[74]

Heat reaches the body in two ways: conduction through the skin and lip of the bamboo, and radiation from the base. Some interesting research has hypothesised that the particular wavelength of light from burning moxa may have special resonances with the signalling systems in the body, thus opening up the possibility that moxibustion works on another entirely different level of signalling than is currently understood. Readers should check out Merlin Young's comprehensive book about moxibustion, *The Moon over Matsushima*, for more inspiration here.[75]

Finally, there are effects that emerge when deploying Manaka's meridian frequencies (applying stimulation at specific frequencies of beats per minute) that have both local and systemic effects of releasing tight tissues.

In the light of all of this, we can see that Ontake is a powerful healing tool that seems to communicate with our patients on a surprising number of levels: olfactory, auditory and kinaesthetic. We can now attempt to describe, from a TEAM perspective, what Ontake might be doing.

Moves Stagnation of Qi and Blood

The most obvious effect of this is the rapidity with which tight muscles get softer, often within a few seconds. Swollen areas and contusions also improve rapidly. Indurations on the abdomen can soften with just a few seconds of knocking (percussive tapping with the bamboo).

Improves the Flow of Qi and Blood in *Kyo* Areas

Weak, cold, dry, lustreless skin can improve noticeably within a minute or so. In palpatory terms, this means that if the skin feels rough initially, it should change to

---

74   Auteroche, B. (1992). *Acupuncture and Moxibustion: A Guide to Clinical Practice.* Edinburgh: Churchill Livingstone, p. 88.

75   Young, M. (2012). *The Moon over Matsushima: Insights into Moxa and Mugwort.* United Kingdom: Godiva Books, pp. 236–243.

feeling smooth. This has major implications for the energy flow in these areas and, as we will see, the reflex areas that they control.

Improves Energy

Most recipients report an improvement in energy levels. This ties in to Birch's three-circle model of regulation discussed in chapter 3. As the channel flow improves, the functional systems improve, and thus, overall energy and vitality improve.

Relieves Pain

We all know that warmth is extremely comforting. Put simply, Ontake feels good! Clearly, if tight muscles relax, this can improve pain, but *kyo*-type pains also improve when bamboo is applied locally—for example, on painful shoulders where muscle tone is poor and the skin feels flaccid. Ontake is also spectacularly effective for the rapid release of pain using holographic systems such as those discussed in part 3 of this book.

Calms the Mind and Relaxes the Whole Body

One of the most obvious supplementary effects is a profound sense of relaxation during treatment. This is undoubtedly a function of the heat from the bamboo but may also be connected to the hypnotic ticking of the metronome. It is for this reason that it is essential to use natural ticking sounds on the metronome, rather than electronic beeping sounds, as well as low volume during treatment. Otherwise, these subliminal benefits can be lost.

By combining a number of modalities, Ontake seems to affect both deficiency and excess, regulating qi and blood. It is very relaxing and calms the mind.

Contraindications

Ontake has a physical effect on the tissues when applied with methods such as rolling or knocking, but at its core, it is a moxibustion technique. Moxibustion is the combustion of *mogusa*, the dried "punk" or wool made from the leaves of *Artemisia vulgaris*, commonly known as mugwort. There is a vast range of moxibustion techniques, categorised as direct or indirect methods, which are applied directly on or over the skin. Indirect methods include burning moxa on the end of the needle, dragging large moxa boxes across the back, and lighting moxa cigars that provide radiant heat.

There are also methods for rolling moxa wool into cones, both large and small. These can be burnt directly on the skin or with an intermediary, such as a slice of ginger. As the bamboo acts as an intermediary between the burning moxa and the skin, we can categorise Ontake as indirect moxibustion, but the bamboo also makes firm contact with the tissues, making it slightly unusual: a heated, pressing, and tapping tool.

Many substances other than mugwort can provide heat in TEAM. In TCM, infrared lamps are commonly used instead of traditional moxibustion, which is time-consuming to perform. In addition to these modern methods, heat can be applied by burning sulphur, wax, tobacco, mulberry wood, peach wood, and rush pith.[76] Ontake is therefore entering a crowded field about which much has been written.

What are the contraindications for moxa in general, and can we extend these to Ontake? Are the contraindications different in Chinese and Japanese traditions? Below is a table with information taken from two sources, one TCM and one JAM. I have grouped these contraindications into broad categories that enable comparison and discussion.

Table 8: Contraindications and Considerations in Classical Moxibustion Theory

Category	TCM CONTRAINDICATIONS [76]	JAM CONTRAINDICATIONS [77]
Hot or Excess Conditions	Febrile diseases Deficiency heat conditions Excess heat conditions Liver excess headaches	Patients with very high fever Serious cases (severely debilitated)
Stroke	Spastic stroke	
Exhaustion	Severe weakness	Extreme fatigue

---

76 Auteroche, B. (1992). *Acupuncture and Moxibustion: A Guide to Clinical Practice.* Edinburgh: Churchill Livingstone.

77 Birch, S., & Ida J. (1998). Japanese Acupuncture: A Clinical Guide. Brookline: Paradigm Publications.

Overdoing it	Inebriation or satiety after eating too much	When the patient is inebriated, very hungry, or very full Before or after a hot bath or sauna
Anatomical, local, and cosmetic considerations		Do not burn moxa directly on: • Areas of inflammation; instead, treat proximal and distal to the inflammation • Over large blood vessels • Directly over sites of dermatological disease • The face, in case of scarring
Pregnancy		On the lower abdomen on pregnant women
Diabetes		Only moxa diabetic patients on the torso, not the limbs
Children		Use milder techniques on children

In TCM, which is dominated by herbal thinking, moxibustion is considered to be warming and heating. It is therefore indicated for treating cold conditions and (typically) contraindicated for hot conditions. This is simple yin and yang thinking and makes perfect sense from a herbal perspective. In Japanese traditions, however, moxibustion is applied with finer materials that burn at lower temperatures. It is thus considered to be more stimulating than heating, and this means it is used in quite different ways.[78]

Thus, while there are some contraindications that are the same, the Japanese list above is more nuanced, with a pragmatic focus on anatomical areas to avoid and ways to moderate the treatment accordingly.

The problem with listing contraindications for moxibustion is that there are so many ways to apply it that not all of the contraindications apply to all of the methods. Ontake is different than applying a moxa stick and performing small cone moxibustion. Using the broad categories of condition in table 8, can we extrapolate any contraindications for Ontake? Table 9 explores each contraindication category in light of my ten years of clinical practice with Ontake and comes to a verdict on the validity of each.

---

78 Kivity, O. (2018). Japanese Acupuncture and Moxibustion—What's So Unique? *European Journal of Oriental Medicine, 9*(2).

Table 9: Discussion of Contraindications in Relation to Ontake

Category	Discussion	Verdict
Hot or Excess conditions	While there has been some use of small cone moxibustion on DU 14 for fever, there is no clinical research into the use of Ontake. If this kind of condition came my way, I would prefer tried and tested methods rather than Ontake.	Contraindicated for fever
Stroke	The next chapter presents a long case study of a patient with spastic stroke, and I would certainly recommend Ontake for this.	Treatable
Exhaustion	The classical contraindications seem to be for *extreme* fatigue. In milder cases, reducing the dosage of treatment overall is essential.	Treat with caution
Overdoing it	This contraindication makes complete sense for all treatment, not just moxibustion.	Contraindicated
Anatomical, Local and Cosmetic Considerations	Contraindications for treating over enlarged blood vessels, areas of inflammation, and sites of dermatological disease make complete sense for Ontake. It is impossible to sterilise the bamboo if it contacts broken skin and body fluids. If applied sensibly, Ontake is probably the safest method for treating the face with moxa. Areas of inflammation should be avoided, but the borders may be treated.	Contraindicated Apply with care Apply with care
Pregnancy	Ontake is extremely useful in pregnancy, both for the rapid relief of pain and to calm the mind.	Apply with care Avoid the waist and sacrum in the first four months.
Diabetes	The heat from normal use of Ontake is not enough to burn the skin and therefore not a risk for diabetics.	No risk
Children	Ontake can definitely be used with children, but with a much-reduced dose.	Apply with care

From this discussion we can now make a list of contraindications and cautions specific to Ontake.

Ontake should not be applied:
- In grave cases of febrile disease
- Over broken skin
- Over areas where bloodletting was just applied (If exposed to blood, the bamboo should be thrown away.)
- Over areas of inflammation
- When the patient is intoxicated with alcohol or drugs
- If the patient has eaten too much or is very hungry
- One hour before or after a hot bath or sauna

Caution should be applied when treating:
- Children
- Pregnant women
- Inflammation
- The face

Summary

Ontake works on many levels, not just through radiant and conducted heat, but also on mechanical, auditory, olfactory and rhythmic levels. It calms the mind.

Through the lens of clinical practice, we can extrapolate what contraindications might apply to Ontake from the general contraindications for moxibustion and construct a list of pragmatic dos and don'ts that inform safe practice.

The chapters ahead explore four main areas of application for Ontake:
1. Root Treatment—whole-body root treatments using Ontake alone
2. Branch Treatment:
   a. Ontake for specific conditions
   b. Ontake for pain relief using holographic models
3. Supplementary Treatment—additional regulation through the Hirata zones

We start this exploration by examining how we can use Ontake to treat the root.

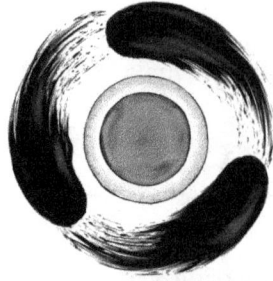

CHAPTER 8

ROOT TREATMENT

Introducing two whole-body root treatments.

Working on the whole body is a good way to practise. It will quickly get you familiar with the techniques and may well give you some surprising results.

Non-Pattern-Based Root Treatments with Bamboo

Most of the applications for Ontake in this book are concerned with *hyochiho* branch treatment, and in the limited literature in Japanese and English, its application has only been discussed in this context. If bamboo is used primarily to address symptoms, what do we do when faced with a patient with multiple symptoms? Do we add a little bit of bamboo for one symptom, treat a bit more for the next and continue until we have covered them all?

If we left this decision to our patients, the answer would be "Yes, certainly! Please don't stop!" If you had asked Dr Manaka or Kodo Fukushima, the founder of the Toyohari Association, the answer to this would have been a resounding "*Chigau!*" ("No way!"). As we will see in chapter 10 on dosage, patients with multiple symptoms tend to be frailer than patients with one or a few symptoms. In these cases, it makes much more sense to treat at a root level, rather than attempting to treat the multiple expressions of root imbalance manifesting in the branch. In fact, we will see that chasing and treating multiple symptoms can have adverse outcomes.

Nevertheless, if Fukushima defined acupuncture as "the differentiation of *kyo* and *jitsu* followed by the application of *ho* and *sha*", could we not apply Ontake over the whole body with the same intention, balancing *kyu* and *jitsu* with *ho* and *sha*?[79]

If we consider the models of the body discussed in chapter 3, namely, Manaka's octahedron or Birch's three-circle model of distortions, we can see that applying bamboo over the whole body could have significant effects, either in balancing the octahedron or in correcting the distortions. These effects would be at the root level, affecting the core energy of the body.

If we applied such a treatment, what form would it take? What would such a whole-body treatment achieve, and for what conditions could it be used? How long should such a treatment take? To answer these questions, we need to look at existing root treatment concepts and understand what elements we should draw from them to treat at this level with bamboo.

Pattern Recognition

In acupuncture, most root treatments are dependent on pattern recognition. For example, in TCM we identify patterns of deficiency and excess, such as liver yin deficiency or liver fire blazing. In Meridian Therapy or *Toyohari*, we identify a primary *sho*, such as spleen *kyo*, with a secondary *sho*, such as liver *jitsu*. In Manaka treatment, we identify structural patterns relating to the Eight Extraordinary Vessels, such as the Yin Qiao/Ren Mai pair.

In all these examples, the treatment that is applied must fit the pattern identified. This means that for liver fire blazing, we must use points that quell liver fire, and this selection should differ from those that nourish yin.

There is, however, a tradition in acupuncture, and especially in moxibustion, of giving generalised treatments that do not depend on pattern identification. Perhaps the most famous of these in moxibustion is the Sawada protocol, "a formula of points that could be used on all patients, regardless of complaint or condition. This formula fortified the patient's constitution and strengthened the qi and the defensive and healing energies".[80]

---

79   Fukushima, K. (1991). *Meridian Therapy*. Tokyo: Toyo Hari Medical Association, p. 148.

80   Manaka, Y., Itaya, K., & Birch, S. (1995). *Chasing the Dragon's Tail: The Theory and Practice of Acupuncture in the Work of Yoshio Manaka*. Brookline: Paradigm Publications, p. 177.

Developed by Japanese moxibustion practitioner Ken Sawada (1877–1938), this was known as Sawada's *taiji* moxa treatment (*taikyoku* in Japanese*)*, a whole-body treatment that could be administered to all, with a broad formula of points that were applied depending on pressure pain, not theory.

Sawada's assistant Bunshi Shirota (1900–1974) later developed a simpler version of the *taiji* moxa treatment, and naturally, Manaka designed two himself, one for moxibustion and one for needling with ion-pumping cords, both of which incorporated his structural ideas about the octahedron.

Another precedent for a whole-body treatment that is not dependent on diagnosis or pattern recognition comes from Shonishin, a style of paediatric channel stimulation from Japan for infants and children up to seven years old. This treatment is administered by stroking or tapping the channels with specialised metal tools, focusing predominantly on the yang aspects of the body, as well as the *yangming* channels on the anterior torso. The order of treatment goes from arms to legs, then chest, abdomen, back, and back of the legs.

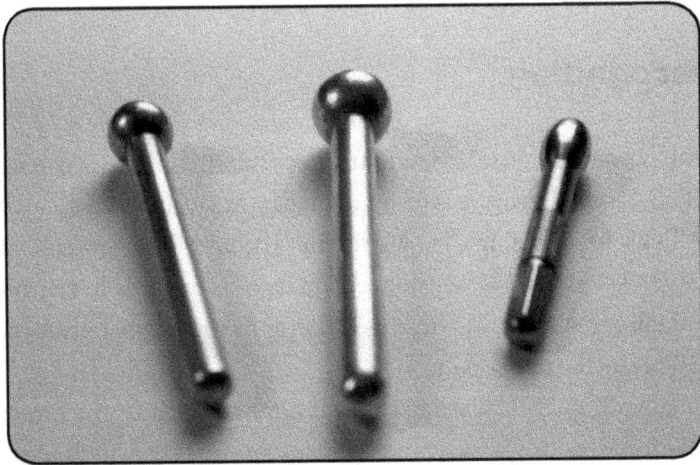

Rounded copper, silver and stainless steel *enshin* used
for stroking the channels on children.

Introducing this core treatment approach for children in his book *Shonishin: Japanese Pediatric Acupuncture*, Stephen Birch coined the term "core non-pattern-based root treatment" (NPBRT). This accurately describes a root treatment approach that can be used with Ontake: a whole-body treatment with systemic effects that can be applied to all, without the need for pattern identification and modification according to pattern.[81]

81　Birch, S. (2016). *Shonishin Japanese Pediatric Acupuncture*. Stuttgart: Thieme, p. 48.

Treating Channels Not Points

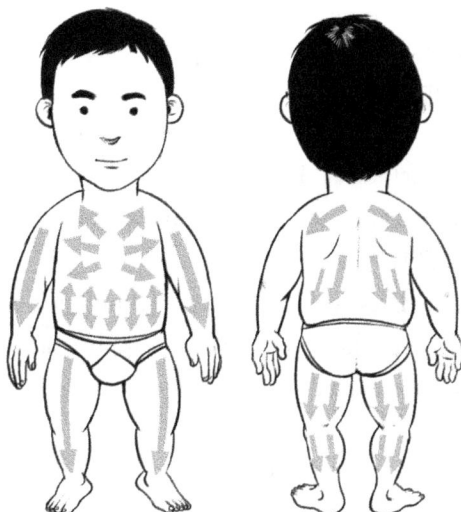

Stroking zones for Shonishin treatment.

What is notable about the Shonishin NPBRT is that it does not involve treating acupuncture points, prioritising instead stroking or pressing along whole channels. This is not unique to Shonishin. Canada-based moxibustion specialist Junji Mizutani described a case where he used *oshi kyu* press moxibustion, pressing with a moxa stick along all the yang channels on a patient with constipation, who was very yang deficient and cold.[82]

This case captured my imagination many years before I came across Ontake. The press moxa was applied to the acupuncture channels, not the points. As we will see throughout this book, bamboo is a remarkably mobile and agile tool that can be applied and moved anywhere along a channel. This case always stuck in my mind, leading me to study and practise *oshi kyu*, and was one of the inspirations for the techniques presented later in this chapter.

Another example of treating channels rather than points comes from a description of a TCM acupuncture technique with a cutaneous needle (*pi fu zhen*). Auteroche described whole-body treatments with a cutaneous needle:

> For diseases of the organs, treatment should start with 'primary tapping'.
> Whatever the disease, this technique consists of tapping along the inner bladder

---

82   Mizutani, J. (1998). *Practical Moxibustion Therapy*. Canada: North American Journal of Oriental Medicine.

line, on either side of the spine, starting from the shoulders and moving to the lumbosacral area. This is done downwards and upwards three times...

After primary tapping, points are chosen according to which organ is implicated in the disease. Examples:

- Diseases of the respiratory system apply stimulation between the 1st and 7th thoracic vertebrae (T-1–T-7)
- Diseases of the nervous system and psychological diseases: apply tapping to T-3 and L-2 as well as the head
- Diseases of the digestive system: apply stimulation between T-7 and L-5
- Diseases of the genitourinary system: apply stimulation between L-5 and the sacral vertebrae.[83]

In this description, in all cases, the inner bladder line is tapped with the needle, and this constitutes the primary treatment, with different areas emphasised for different conditions. The "primary tapping" is first applied to everyone, regardless of the presentation. Following this, there is some treatment variation according to the location of the symptoms.

Even with cupping therapy, there are protocols for an NPBRT for generalised wellness. Dr Manaka described a general health maintenance approach for lay practitioners using cupping.[84]

From the examples above, we can see there is precedent to treat at the root level without pattern recognition and by stimulating acupuncture channels rather than points. Of course, within the bodywork community that uses the qi paradigm, this is a given. In Tui Na and Shiatsu, stimulation of the whole channel is the norm. It may be true to say, however, that in recent years, the influence of TCM in the West on Shiatsu training has led to the penetration of acupressure point prescription protocols into channel-based Zen Shiatsu, something really quite alien to the original Japanese therapy.[85]

---

83   Auteroche, B. (1992). *Acupuncture and Moxibustion: A Guide to Clinical Practice.* Edinburgh: Churchill Livingstone, pp. 94–95.

84   Birch, S., & Ida, J. (1998) *Japanese Acupuncture: A Clinical Guide.* Brookline: Paradigm Publications, p. 208.

85   Kivity, O., (2018). Japanese Acupuncture and Moxibustion—What's So Unique? *European Journal of Oriental Medicine, 9*(2).

Whole-Body Treatments with Bamboo

In the timeline of acupuncture, Ontake is a brand-new therapy. Within the timeline of bamboo treatment itself, its combined use with Manaka's frequencies is even more recent. There is almost no literature on this. Thus, developing a whole-body treatment required integrating the precedents of whole-body treatments from other modalities, as well as a willingness to experiment with basic acupuncture principles.

Guidelines

Below are two NPBRT routines with Ontake that I have developed over the last ten years. Although different in approach, they both share one critical rule of application—namely, that treatment must be short and quick. As we will see in later chapters, Ontake treatment seems very innocuous. It's warm, it's relaxing, and it feels nice. In fact, Ontake is deceptively gentle.

If we go back to the doorbell analogy of chapter 3, Ontake sends signals on many levels with heat, sound, the frequencies themselves, and its percussive physical action on the soft tissue. Even the smell of moxa is a trigger. This is like ringing on the doorbell, knocking on the door, and singing Christmas carols all at the same time. Grandma is definitely getting up from her chair to open the door, but if you carry on like this for too long, she's not going to be too happy by the time she gets there! Thus, it's crucial to keep a whole-body treatment with bamboo light and quick: the duration should not exceed twenty-five minutes on a robust patient and should be even shorter on someone weak. This concept of limiting treatment and dosage is explored in detail in chapter 10.

Many of the instructions in this book suggest strokes to use in certain places. These are guidelines only, and you can safely substitute in other strokes. Each person is different, and their individual anatomy suggests different strokes. The arm of a big patient presents at a different height and angle than that of a small patient, and this influences your posture as you treat. Moreover, patients' muscle tones vary. Both of these factors suggest different techniques to treat the same channel. Sometimes you'll be drawn to press on a channel, and at other times, particularly as you get familiar with the strokes, you'll be drawn to a different technique, such as rolling. Sometimes you'll choose to tap slowly, and at other times, rapidly in double time. Thus, there are no rules with bamboo, except that the stroke should feel comfortable both to you and to the patient. You are the best judge of which stroke to use where.

Eyes and Nose

Tapping techniques with the base of the bamboo are great on flat areas such as the limbs or back. On the face, various protruding structures can insert themselves into the smouldering, concave mouth with unfortunate consequences. The eye is convex, so you must never touch it with the lighted end of the bamboo. The nose should only be treated with the side of the bamboo. This rule also applies to the chin, ear lobes and prominent cheekbones. All these areas can be treated, of course, but with the side of the bamboo, not the lighted mouth.

After Treatment

Encourage your patients to drink a lot of water. Ontake whole-body treatments are hot, moving and yang, so the body needs fluids as it processes the changes.

Bamboo Max—A Non-Pattern-Based Root Treatment

This sequence was the first of the whole-body treatments to be developed and was based loosely on the Shonishin sequence taught by Stephen Birch. I also like to think of it as a *yangming* sequence, as there is arguably more focus on the large intestine and stomach channel than others.

The sequence is divided into two sections, with the patient lying first supine and then prone. The sequence in the prone position can be given on its own and is nicknamed "Bamboo Mini plus legs". Bamboo Mini, simply working on the back, is also beneficial as an adjunctive end treatment to a standard acupuncture session.

Aim

The goal of this strong tonic treatment is to create a broad range of effects: increase energy, relax tight muscles, relieve stress and harmonise digestion.

Start with a general tension assessment of the arms, shoulders, hips, and legs. This tension assessment gives you valuable feedback about the dynamic effects of the treatment. After each step of the treatment, you can re-palpate or recheck at the feedback areas mentioned. [86]

---

86   For videos of how these areas are treated, visit The Ontake Channel on YouTube and look under the Practical playlist: https://www.youtube.com/theontakechannel

Routine

1. Work along the three arm yang channels from hand to shoulders on both sides, large intestine (108), triple burner (152), and small intestine (120). For the small intestine, lift the arm so the patient's hand is at the opposite shoulder, exposing the back of the arm.

   Feedback Areas: top of the trapezius, neck mobility.

2. Starting at the thigh, work your way down the stomach channel (132). Work your way up the spleen channel on the anterior medial aspect of the leg (132), stopping slightly above SP 10.

   Feedback Areas: top of the trapezius, neck mobility, abdominal tension, shoulder tension and range of movement.

3. Touch and close or roll the whole abdomen (132). Press or lean in a circle around the navel, and knock on indurations or stubborn tight points at the appropriate frequency.

   Feedback Areas: abdominal tension, upper- and mid-back tightness.

4. Turn the head to one side and tap or roll the side of the neck (120). Repeat on the other side.

5. Tap and close over the inguinal groove until it feels softer (132 or 120).

   Feedback Areas: tension in the inguinal groove, lower back (reach hands underneath patient to palpate lumbar region).

Steps 4 and 5 are explained in more detail in chapter 12.

Turn the patient over and perform steps 1–12 of Bamboo Mini plus legs.

Bamboo Mini Plus Legs

The following sequence can be divided into two distinct sections, which can be performed separately. Bamboo Mini comprises steps 1–7 and the leg sequence comprises steps 8–13.

Tops of the shoulders

1. The shoulders are mostly covered by the gall bladder and small intestine channels, which respond to 120 beats per minute. Tap the scapula and trapezius lightly with the mouth of the bamboo (120). As this is a broad area,

it can be useful (and soothing) to tap in double time. If very *kyo*, touch and close.

2. Roll the same area, focusing on and adapting your depth and strength to the areas of *kyo* and *jitsu* (120).

3. If the top of the traps remains stiff, try rolling at 152. Vibrating or bouncing can be very useful here. If the traps still don't relax, treat SI 9, 10 and especially SI 11 in the infraspinous fossa (120).

4. Tap the bladder channel on either side of the spine (112). Some people find it easier to work from T-1 to T-7 first and then proceed to the lower points. Others like to connect the whole back in one long sequence.

5. Roll lightly on *kyo* areas and firmly on *jitsu* (112). Lean on especially *jitsu* areas for four or eight beats, and then roll afterwards.

6. For urinary, gynaecological, and sacral problems, roll over the sacrum (104). Standing on lower Du Mai points for one bar is very relaxing. Stand the bamboo below L-2 for one bar, below L-3 for another, below L-4 for another, and continue.

7. Treat *kubi koshi* reactions in a line on the waist from below the ribs to the top of the ASIS.
   Feedback Area: the back of the neck. Kubi koshi *is discussed in chapter 12.*

8. Use super-knocking in double time from the buttock to calf, first over the bladder (112) then over the gall bladder channel (120).

9. Press, knock, and roll down the back of the calf, releasing *jitsu* areas (112). Lean on especially tight areas for four or eight beats.

10. If there is tension on the medial or lateral sides of the calf, treat there (120).

11. Roll up and down on the sole of the feet, starting at the lateral aspect and working your way medially (120).

12. Press the pads of each toe for four beats (120).

13. The Japanese insomnia point in the centre of the heel and KID-1 are both useful points to treat. Hold the bamboo at the centre of the plantar side of the heel for eight beats (120). Hold on KID-1, about two thirds of the way down the sole for eight beats (120). As this is the end of the treatment, an excellent way to close is to turn off the metronome and warm these points in silence.

Duration and Dosage

Bamboo Max should take no more than twenty-five minutes in total to perform, though naturally, a session takes longer if we include bookend processes like chatting, getting changed, routine diagnosis, and palpation. Bamboo Max is designed as a full-body root treatment; therefore, additional root treatment with other modalities is redundant, and branch treatment should be added with caution about the overall dosage.

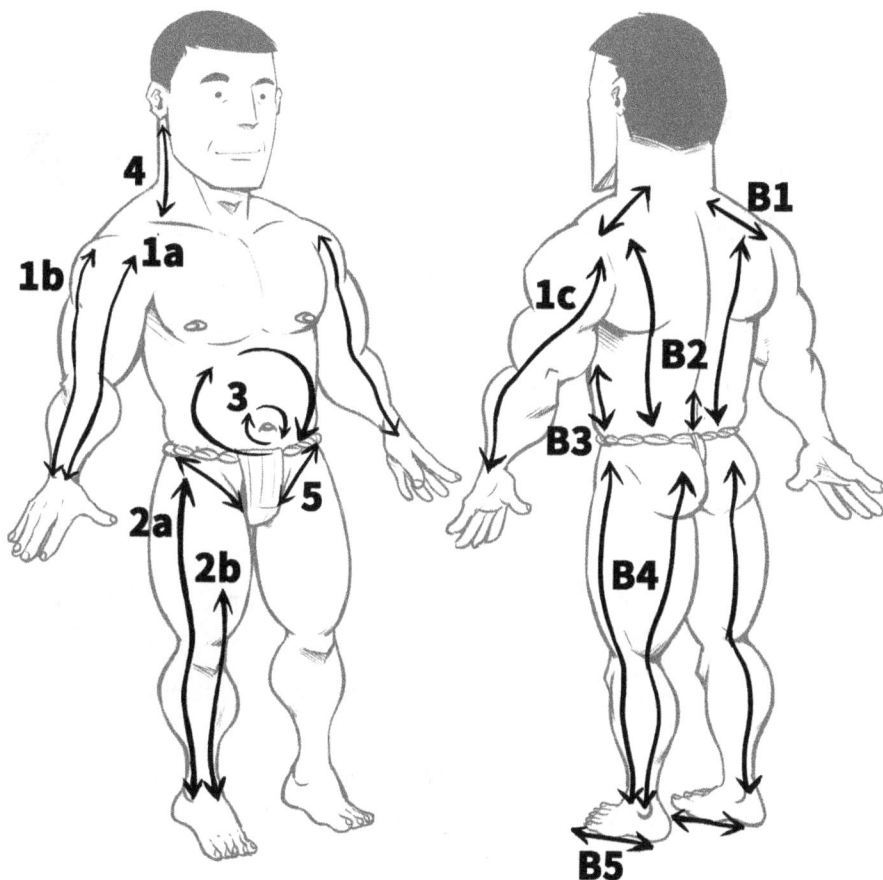

Bamboo Max (1-5) and Bamboo Mini plus Legs (B1-B5).

Table 10 Bamboo Max Summary (25–30 min.)

	Area	Frequency
1a 1b 1c	Arms, (LI, TH, SI)	108, 152, 120
2a 2b	Legs, front (ST, SP)	132
3	Abdomen	132
4	Side of neck	120

5	Inguinal groove	132 or 120
B1	Shoulder (GB) If stubborn add TB (152) or LI (108)	120
B1	Shoulder blade (SI)	120
B2	Upper back (BL)	112
B2	Lower back (BL)	112
B2	Sacrum (Du Mai)	104
B3	*Kubi koshi* (sides of the abdomen)	120
B4	Buttocks and legs, posterior and lateral aspects (BL, GB)	112/120
B5	Sole (KID)	120
B5	Toes	120

Cases

Male: Late 50s. Stress Symptoms.

Our clinic had just finished doing a fundraising drive using Bamboo Max exclusively, with four practitioners donating the receipts from our bamboo sessions to our favourite charity for feeding the homeless. This Singaporean businessman was visiting Kuala Lumpur and heard from a friend that Bamboo Max was very relaxing.

On his first session, he arrived late, feeling stressed and with a full-blown migraine. Bamboo Max was applied without pattern diagnosis. At the end of the session, he had to be woken up and found he no longer had a migraine. We encouraged him to drink plenty of water, and he left, feeling refreshed.

He returned a second time a few months later, this time with severe gastric pain. Once again, he woke up after the session, feeling much relieved.

Another few months passed until he was back in town, this time with back pain, wanting bamboo. At this point, our practice manager took me to the side and asked if we shouldn't be encouraging him to have acupuncture, as his was a complicated case needing fuller diagnosis and treatment. But the patient already had so much faith in the bamboo that I was happy to repeat this basic root treatment. Once again, he felt great relief.

In total, he came in five times over a year and a half, each time with a severe stress-related symptom, and he left "feeling cured" each time. This experience taught me that bamboo could be used very simply to "ring the doorbell" and trigger the body to correct itself. Moreover, this kind of root treatment can benefit a wide variety of conditions without complicated differential diagnosis or any focus on symptom management. In its way, it's a *taiji* Ontake treatment.

Female: 39. Fibromyalgia.

The vibrations from go-karting with her kids triggered some neck pain. It kept getting worse until finally, presenting with fatigue, whole body pain, and weakness, she was diagnosed with fibromyalgia in 2009 and decided to come for acupuncture.

At first, treatment was primarily with Toyohari, which kept the symptoms at bay and improved her quality of life. In late 2011, it seemed the acupuncture was no longer as effective, and she quit for a while to try medicating with Lyrica. This proved disastrous, and in early 2012 she returned worse than ever before. She was unable to walk, sit, or talk without feeling exhausted. Her pulse was extremely weak, thin, rapid, and floating. Amid concerns about over-dosage of Lyrica and liver toxicity (she also had subcostal pain), treatment began with a very short Bamboo Max. She improved dramatically and contacted her doctor to stop treatment with Lyrica. Since then, Bamboo Max has been the only treatment given, and she has maintained an excellent quality of life with little pain and greatly enhanced energy.

It's interesting to note that although she had a typical deficiency heat pulse, warm bamboo on the yang channels consolidated and strengthened the pulse and also addressed her symptoms. In other words, working on the yang channels with heat strengthened the yin.

Female: 40. Neck Pain and Tinnitus.

After teaching this routine in Brazil in mid-2019, I was approached on the second day of the workshop by one of the students who had been the model in her group. She wanted to report that her long-term tinnitus had reduced dramatically after Bamboo Max. In my experience, tinnitus is often linked to neck and shoulder issues, and when I enquired about this, she confirmed that she had long-term chronic neck pain. This too had reduced in intensity. I include this case because tinnitus is such a difficult problem to treat with acupuncture, but in this single instance, it responded unexpectedly to a mere thirty minutes of Ontake.

BB-8—An Alternative Root Treatment

Manaka's Octahedral model as it relates to the Eight Extras is explored in more detail in chapter 12. If we want to treat the Eight Extras directly with Ontake, only the Ren and Du Mai have their own trajectories, points, and frequencies. The remaining extra vessels use or "borrow" points on the twelve main channels. In classical acupuncture, to access them, we treat individual points, such as KID 9, to affect the Yin Wei Mai, or more commonly, we treat the master and coupled points of each vessel.

However, some commentators say, when using any points of *taiyang*, not just SI 3 and BL 62, we are still at some level, accessing the Du Mai and the Yang Qiao Mai. For example, when treating neck pain with Toyohari, copper and zinc are usually applied to SI 3 and BL 62, but point variations can be tried if the results are not satisfactory, such as SI 7 and BL 59.[87] If this is the case, then treating the channels of the master and coupled points with bamboo may also access the related Eight Extra. Indeed, this principle can be exploited for treating stubborn reactions during step 1 of Manaka's treatment method (see chapter 13).

This thought led to the development of Bamboo-8 (BB-8, for Star Wars fans), a simple tapping routine that not only targets Ren, Dai and Du Mai by tapping on their accessible pathways, but also involves the whole octahedron created by the Eight Extras by tapping on the channels related to the master and coupled points.

As usual, tap briskly and lightly to activate the whole channel pathway. The treatment ends with a familiar back sequence with the emphasis on the midline. Treatment duration should be no more than twenty-five minutes.

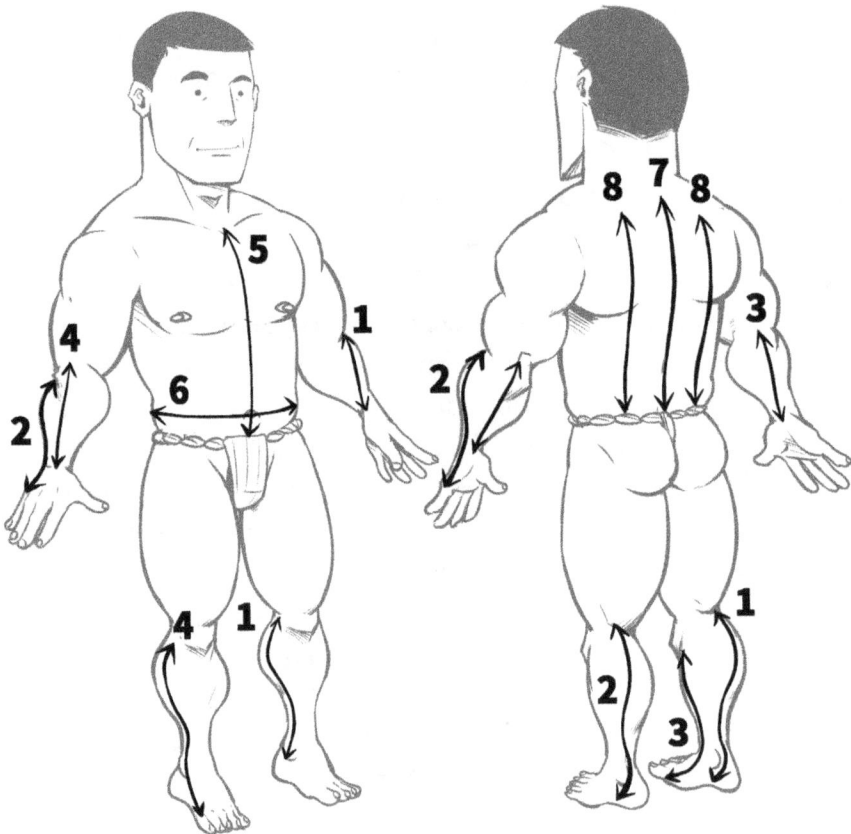

The BB-8 Sequence.

87   Kivity, O. (Ed.) (2007). Kikei Nuggets, *Keiraku Chiryo – International Toyohari News*, p. 39.

Table 11 BB-8 Sequence

	VESSEL	CHANNELS	TREATMENT AREA	BPM
1.	Yin Qiao Ren Mai	Lung, kidney	LU 5 to LU 9 KID 6 to KID 10	126 120
2.	Yang Qiao Du Mai	Small intestine, bladder	SI 3 to SI 8 BL 40 to BL 62	120 112
3.	Yin Wei Chong Mai	Pericardium, spleen	P 3 to P 7 SP 4 to SP 10	176 132
4.	Yang Wei Dai Mai	Triple burner, gall bladder	TB 5 to TB 10 GB 34 to GB 42	152 120
5.	Ren Mai	Anterior midline	REN 2 to REN 22	104
6.	Dai Mai	Horizontal Band at Navel	KID 16, ST 25, SP 15, GB 26	132 120
7. 8.	Du Mai	Posterior midline, Bladder	DU 14 to DU 2, BL 11 to BL 26	104 112

This routine cycles between treating yin and yang channels on the hand and foot, sequentially. As with Bamboo Max, after treating the arms and legs, attention is focused first on the abdomen and then on the back.

Case

Female: 35. Labour Induction

In this very unusual case, the patient went into labour with strong contractions, which were getting more intense and more frequent, and she was admitted to a hospital about ten days before her due date. After a few hours, the contractions, which were not Braxton Hicks, stopped. At this point, she decided to stay in the hospital because she didn't want to go home to her husband. She then booked an acupuncture labour induction and arrived still wearing her hospital tag.

It took some time for us to unravel the situation in the first consultation. Not only was she in a very stressful position with her husband, but she had intense back pain and sciatica. Initial treatments were standard labour induction points and Ontake over the lung channel to relieve the back pain (see chapter 10 for an explanation).

She returned three days later. Her back was somewhat better, but she had had no contractions. By now her doctor had given her a deadline for chemical induction, so she felt under even more pressure. Treatment was repeated with the addition of small cone moxibustion at SP 6 and BL 67, and Ontake around the waist.

The next day, there still were no contractions, so we took a different approach and did BB-8, mostly with her sitting and working around the ASIS and sacrum instead of tapping on Ren and Dai Mai. This had an instant effect on her back pain and seemed to change her mood.

The next day we repeated BB-8. Once again, she felt much calmer, her pain was now quite minor, and a day later she took the time to text us that she was going into labour.

In other contexts, BB-8 seems to be very effective for back pain, perhaps because it reorganises the flow of qi in the eight quadrants sequentially. It is also very calming. This case shows that sometimes—particularly when stress, resentment, and stagnation are involved—it is better to think outside the box, focusing on the root, in this case with a NPBRT.

Summary

This chapter describes two tapping routines to use on patients, either solely for relaxation, or for the treatment of diverse symptoms by addressing the root. This kind of root treatment can be used:

- With a very complicated presentation where there are many symptoms
- When the patient is weak and you want to build her energy
- When you are simply not sure of the diagnosis and how to proceed
- When the patient has arrived late and time is short

Bamboo Max has been used by more practitioners over a longer time than BB-8, but I have found BB-8 to be equally effective as a simple root treatment. In the next chapter, we will look at the other wheel on the axle: branch treatment, or how to treat symptoms.

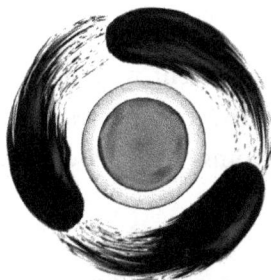

CHAPTER 9

BRANCH TREATMENT

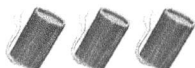

Using Ontake to treat a wide variety of symptoms.

In Chinese medicine, treatment is based on both disease and pattern diagnosis. Any time therapy is applied, whether it is herbal medicine, acupuncture, moxibustion, or bloodletting, the provider should have a clear idea of the pattern of disharmony, causing the disease manifestation. Previously in this book, bloodletting as a therapeutic intervention, especially related to blood stasis patterns, has been looked at almost as if it were to be applied in a vacuum or as a monotherapy. However, clinicians will most likely utilize bloodletting alongside other interventions.

—Henry McCann[88]

Introductory Thoughts

This quotation from *Pricking the Vessels,* Henry McCann's excellent book on bloodletting, can be extended to summarise the role of bamboo in the clinic. Although we have talked much about root treatment—that is, adjusting imbalances

---

88   McCann, H. (2014). *Pricking the Vessels: Bloodletting Therapy in Chinese Medicine.* London: Singing Dragon, p. 121.

in the body as a whole—root treatment with bamboo is a rarity used by very few. Almost all contemporary use of bamboo relates to its effectiveness as a tool to treat the branch, or individual symptoms. Manaka discussed root and branch treatment in the following way:

> In the root treatment, a common pattern is discriminated with the aim of balancing the body as a whole and a common point selection strategy is used regardless of the complaint or disease. If the root treatment is fully successful, specific complaints or localised pain are resolved without symptomatic or local treatment. (At least, that is the way it is supposed to work.) Today both aspects of treatment are considered necessary, like two wheels on an axle.[89]

Manaka's axle analogy is useful to emphasise the mutual importance of treating root and branch but less clear when you consider the order in which to do so. Unless there is something very wrong with the vehicle, both wheels advance together simultaneously. In clinical practice, do you do root treatment before, after, or simultaneously with branch treatment? Manaka emphasised that his main focus was on root treatment, and he preferred to do it first, before branch treatment. This is because doing root treatment creates order when the system is in disarray. Once the system is more ordered, it is easier to do branch treatment.[90]

Additionally, from a practitioner's point of view, starting with root treatment and continuing to symptom relief creates a different kind of order—a useful structure and routine for each session. This is like doing a kata in martial arts. Doing the same thing repeatedly leads to learning and mastery. Having a sequence and order is particularly useful with patients who have multiple symptoms clamouring for attention. Both in Manaka Style Acupuncture (MSA) and Toyohari, the root treatment quite often takes care of several symptoms, leaving only the most stubborn to be addressed by branch treatment. In rare cases, however, in Toyohari, practitioners may start with branch treatment when the patient is in such severe pain that they are not really in a place to receive root treatment.[91]

If we consider the implications of the above in the context of bamboo as a branch treatment, then we can infer two principles:

- Bamboo is rarely applied alone.
- Bamboo is often applied after the root treatment.

---

89   Manaka, Y., (2009). The Concept of Meridians from a Systems Perspective. *NAJOM Special Issue: In Memory of Dr Manaka Yoshio*, 16(47), p. 28.

90   Ibid.

91   Kivity O. (Ed.). (2007). Kikei Nuggets. *Keiraku Chiryo – International Toyohari News*, p. 39.

The beauty of bamboo as a clinical tool is that it integrates with any style of acupuncture. Once you have achieved your main objective of regulating qi and blood in your own particular style, bamboo is a highly adaptable adjunctive treatment that can be added when necessary. This kind of bamboo branch treatment should come towards the end of treatment, or at least after the main mechanisms of root treatment have been put in place. For example, in MSA, the first step involves applying needles connected with ion-pumping cords. This step takes between five and fifteen minutes, and during this time, it can be helpful to apply bamboo for branch treatment.

This chapter explores various symptoms or conditions that have responded well to bamboo branch treatment, including treating painful conditions by treating locally. Historically, Makoto Yamashita and Hideo Shinma have used bamboo for pain relief by applying it at the site of pain. There are, however, other ways of treating pain by applying bamboo distally, and these methods, applied with holographic imaging, are discussed in much detail in the next chapter.

General Principles of Treatment

Bamboo treatment is based on traditional acupuncture principles of balancing yin and yang, specifically *kyojitsu* (deficiency-excess). It uses the application of heat, pressure, and percussion at the channel frequencies to accomplish this. It can, therefore, be used for symptom relief for a wide range of problems.

The most important thing to remember when using bamboo is that it feels good! Letting go of any theoretical considerations, the rhythmic application of warmth feels extremely comforting. When addressing symptoms with bamboo, there are three basic principles to bear in mind:

- Treat locally (where the issue is) by identifying the problem channel or channels and then rolling or tapping at the appropriate frequency.
- Extend the area of treatment outwards laterally and longitudinally from the problem area to balance areas of *kyojitsu* in the problem channel and adjacent ones.
- Add additional distal acupuncture points or areas known to target the problem.

Acupuncturists usually focus on reactive points when needling, but with bamboo, it is more helpful to focus on balancing excess and deficient areas along the channels and affected regions. This means palpating, assessing, and treating whole areas and channels rather than focusing on points. As mentioned in chapter 5, this requires a more engaged kind of palpation, treating what you find, not just at the level of the problem, but also above and below it. This kind of palpation starts to uncover relationships between body areas that are not immediately apparent from established channel theory.

Crunchy Crystals

When rolling on bony areas, you may feel a "crunching" sensation, as if there are crystals between the skin and bone. This sensation is commonly found in reactive areas on the skull, on the dorsum of the feet and hands, and along the medial border of the tibia, but it can manifest along any bony surface. These crunchy areas invariably feel uncomfortable or painful to the patient, and the crystals take more than one treatment to resolve.

The cause of these sensations is a matter of conjecture. The idea that impurities settle as crystal formations in the feet is one of the central concepts of foot reflexology, which aims to break up these deposits. In my practice, I have found this kind of reaction is not limited to the lower part of the body and can even be found on top of the head.

Gout is caused by high levels of uric acid forming urate crystals in the joints, typically causing pain in the big toe but potentially any joint in the body. Another possible explanation is calcium deposits. Pseudogout, or calcium pyrophosphate dihydrate crystal deposition disease (CPDD), is associated with acute and chronic arthritis, and the crystals can form in periarticular areas as well as in the joints themselves.[92]

In a healthy person, is it possible that this sensation of crunchiness is a precursor sign of asymptomatic calcium or urate deposits, often associated with arthritic pain. In a person with existing symptoms of arthritis, these reactions are important to treat.

Whatever the cause, it is important to be gentle when you come to these sensitive areas. Edo wasn't built in a day! It is better to treat a little, often, and lightly than engage in a single comprehensive attempt to eliminate all reactions. Moreover, rolling lightly over a crunchy area for a short time can have significant effects on symptom relief and is a strong clue that you are in an effective treatment area.

Bamboo Mini

Bamboo Max is the whole-body root treatment with bamboo discussed in the previous chapter. Bamboo Mini is the name given to that part of the sequence that focuses on the back. Taken out of context, it is actually a very useful branch treatment for many conditions and is referred to below in several examples.

---

92   Rosales-Alexander, J., Aznar, J. B., & Magro-Checa, C. (2014). Calcium Pyrophosphate Crystal Deposition Disease: Diagnosis and Treatment. *Open Access Rheumatology: Research and Reviews*, 39. DOI:10.2147/oarrr.s39039

Knee Pain

As an example of this approach, it is important to palpate the whole leg from hip to ankle. This immediately focuses your bamboo treatment. It needn't take long. Pick up and squeeze from the top of the thigh to the ankle. Check whether there is tightness in the stomach channel running up to ST 31 and down to ST 37 and ST 39, or whether the tension is more in the calves on the bladder or kidney line. It may be that the main tension is on the gall bladder channel. Sometimes everything feels weak and *kyo,* and there's little or no tightness. Palpating the leg takes a few seconds but immediately narrows your focus so that treating the whole leg with bamboo takes just two to four minutes.

The basic principles are to treat soft and weak areas first with light, warming strokes, such as tapping, touching and closing, light rolling or pressing. Frequently, working on the *kyo* areas releases tighter areas before you come to treat them directly. Recheck, then work on the more *jitsu* areas that remain till they feel more pliable. With these, you would use stronger techniques such as heavier rolling, pressing, leaning or super-knocking.

To treat the knee directly, you can tap around the patella in a circle, connecting stomach and spleen (132). Standing the bamboo or rocking on the eyes of the knee (132) feels comforting and warming. Roll above the knee (132), looking for reactions all the way up to the hip and groin. Check tension along the gall bladder channel and tap, press or roll down from the hip to GB 39 (120). It is important to check for *jitsu* points on the stomach channel from ST 36 to the ankle and press or roll them out until less reactive.

With the patient prone, check the back of the knee and the bladder line on the thigh and calves (112). It may be helpful to treat the lumbar, sacral, and inguinal areas, too. The change in muscle tone should be very rapid, enabling you to treat all of the above in a matter of minutes.

Treating in this way is similar to using acupuncture principles of selecting local, adjacent, and distal points but involves palpating and treating all along the channels. Pain can also be treated using holographic models, such as those of Dr Tan or Hirata. These models are discussed in later chapters.

Conditions

Below is a list of conditions that in my own practice have responded well to bamboo. While not meant to be a definitive list of what can or cannot be treated with bamboo, these treatment suggestions should illustrate ways for you to develop your own routines when treating symptoms. As mentioned above, none of the branch protocols below are standalone treatments. These routines should follow or be integrated concurrently with your preferred root treatment style.

Head

Caution: When working on the head, beware of salient anatomy, such as the eye, nose, and chin, protruding into the concave mouth of the bamboo.

Sinus Problems / Cold / Allergic Rhinitis

In Japanese moxibustion, nasal problems are often treated with moxibustion at tender points on Du Mai, such as DU 22 or DU 23.[93] With bamboo, you can quickly treat more than a single point.

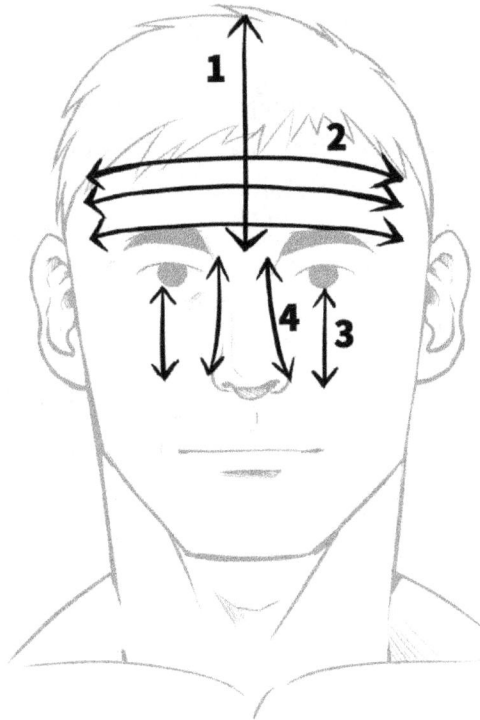

Sinus sequence.

---

93   Shinma, H. (2016). *The Treasure Book of Points Fukaya Kyu*. Tokyo: Hideo Shinma, p. 14; Birch, S., & Ida, J. (1998) *Japanese Acupuncture: A Clinical Guide*. Brookline: Paradigm Publications, p. 127.

Treating Sinus Problems

- Start on the midline of the face between the eyebrows at Yintang and press softly with the side of the bamboo, working your way superiorly to DU 20 and back again, noting any tender areas along the way (104). This feels very relaxing and can be continued for a minute or two.
- Check out the tender areas again and now focus on each one, either rolling slightly harder or gently knocking with the index finger at 104 beats per minute on the side of the bamboo. Knocking on the skull is welcomed by some patients and not tolerated well by others, but in all cases, knock lightly and for a short duration. Follow up with more rolling. By now, the nose should already be feeling clearer.

    It is useful to distinguish between sensations on the skull. Sometimes, the points feel bruised or tender, with a feeling of induration. These points respond well to light knocking and rolling. Other points feel crunchy as if there are crystals underneath the bamboo, reminiscent of a car driving on gravel. These areas respond much better to rolling.

- Touch and close in horizontal lines on the forehead from one side to side to the other at 132 beats per minute or unaccompanied.
- Press or tap from ST 2 to ST 4 (132).
- Press with the side of bamboo on the side of the nose (126 or 108), or sparrow peck with the lighted end without making contact.
- Palpate the large intestine channel and lung channel on the forearm and treat *kyojitsu* there, focusing mainly on tight or painful areas near LI 10 and LU 6.

Upper back points such as BL 11 to 15 are also useful.

Eye Problems

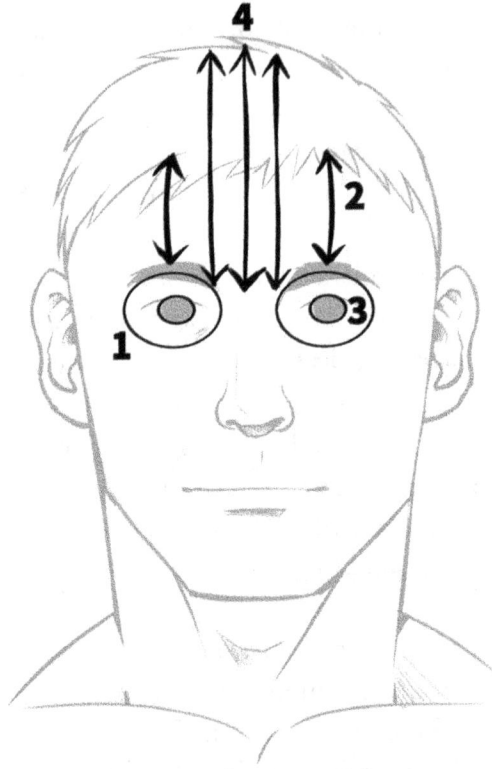

Tapping around the eye.

- Press around the orbit of the eye with the side of the bamboo (108).
- Roll along any crunchy areas you discover along the orbit (108 or channel targeted frequency).
- Roll the forehead along the gall bladder channel (120).
- Cover the eye with a tissue or thin cloth and turn the bamboo on its side. Hold lightly on the eyelid for four beats, above, level with, and below the pupil (108).
- Roll from Yintang to DU 20 along the midline of the head (104) and slightly laterally along the bladder channel (112), focusing on soft or reactive areas.
- Turn the patient over and roll the back of the occiput (112).
- Tap DU 17, just above the occiput until it feels warm (104).
- It may also be useful to treat the neck and shoulders as in the Bamboo Mini treatment or to tap the whole bladder line on the back.

Ear Problems

Many ear problems arise because the circulation of qi and blood is impaired. This can include pain in the ear, tinnitus, or hearing loss. The gall bladder channel makes three broad passes over or around the ear (120). The triple burner channel closely follows the contours of the helix (152). The kidney (120) opens into the ears.

- Palpate for tender or crunchy points along the branches of the gall bladder channel, especially the one encircling the ear, and treat with gentle tapping or rolling (120).
- Press or tap over triple burner around the ear (152).
- Tap directly over the ear, until it feels warm (120).

Repeat all three steps, focusing on painful points between GB 7 and GB 12.

Upper Limb and Back

Shoulder Pain

Shoulder pain typically manifests with areas of deep tension around the shoulder muscles and more distal areas of superficial weakness or deficiency. For example, there may be a deep band of tension from LI 14 to LI 15 and weakness around LI 6 and LI 7. LI8 through LI 10 may also present with tightness.

Palpate the whole arm from shoulder to wrist and note areas of weakness or excess. With the patient lying supine, tap, press, or roll on the affected channels. Supplement the weak areas first, then recheck the tight areas. Palpate for *kyojitsu* on the adjacent channels and treat. When rolling on tight or hard areas, start softly and gradually increase the pressure. If the patient is lying supine, you can lift her elbow and place her hand on the opposite shoulder to expose the back of the arm.

With the patient sitting, roll at DU 14 at the frequencies of the affected channels.

It can be useful to finish with steps 1–4 of the Bamboo Mini. See also the next chapter on pain relief using holographic models.

Case

Female: 49. Neck and Shoulder Pain

Always stressed and frustrated in her work, she developed chronic tension in the shoulders and frequent bouts of neck pain that restricted her range of motion. Usually treated by supplementing lung channel and draining liver channel, she has also responded well to the Bamboo Mini treatment, which leaves her deeply relaxed. Her shoulders are now usually pain-free, but she still gets occasional bouts of neck stiffness. These respond best to tapping at the yang intersection points ST 12 and DU 14 at the appropriate yang channel frequencies.

Wrist Pain and Trigger Finger

As usual, check the whole affected channel for areas of *kyo* and *jitsu*. For example, if someone has pain in the wrist at TB 4, check and treat the whole channel up to the shoulder. Check adjacent channels on both the anterior and posterior surfaces.

With trigger finger, there are likely to be small nodes along the channels that respond to bamboo with focused knocking, leaning, pressing, or rolling. In more severe cases, direct moxa with half-rice-grain cones may be necessary.

Finish with Bamboo Mini, focusing on the upper back, and check the infrascapular fossa and interscapular points for tightness or pressure pain points.

Back Pain

The Bamboo Mini plus legs sequence, the closing part of the Bamboo Max root treatment, can also be used on its own as a branch treatment to address back pain. As it covers the back and legs, it works locally and distally. With the patient prone, work down the body from the shoulders to the ankles.

Bamboo Mini plus legs should take about ten minutes. Focus on problem areas, making sure to treat *kyo* areas lightly and *jitsu* areas more deeply. Super-knocking down the bladder and gall bladder channels on the legs and clearing tension in the medial, posterior, and lateral calf with any appropriate technique works very well. With the patient sitting, roll at DU 14 at the frequencies of the affected channels. When treating pain in the yang channels, DU 14 is often a good place to finish.

The holographic models presented in the next chapter are also essential when treating pain.

Hot Flushes

While it may seem contradictory to use heat to treat hot flushes, a light Bamboo Mini treatment can be helpful. Hot flushes often come with *katakori* (tight shoulders) and cold feet—general indications of counterflow qi, with deficiency below and excess above.

Treatment should focus on the following:
- Release the shoulders and neck.
- Balance the upper and lower by treating the inner bladder line.
- Pull down from the head by treating the legs, especially the soles of the feet.

The Japanese insomnia point *shitsumin*, in the centre of the plantar surface of the heel, and KID 1 are both useful points with which to finish. Stand, rock, or press the bamboo on these points, roll the soles, and press on the plantar surfaces of each toe (120). It feels more soothing to finish the session by turning off the metronome and simply holding the bamboo on KID-1 in silence for a few counts.

Depression and Anxiety

Press down the spine from T-3 to T-9, looking for reactive points in the intervertebral spaces. The five points of the Du Mai from T-3 to T-9 (DU 12 – DU 8) are known as the Upper Back Governor Vessel Five[94] and were used by Fukaya with *okyu* (small cone moxibustion) in all nervous disorders. They are also referred to as Fukaya's neurogenic points or Fukaya's anxiety points. DU 12, in particular, is thought to regulate the nervous system and is often the focus of treatment in Shonishin paediatric treatments with emotionally labile kids.[95] Tetsuya Fukushima, a contemporary proponent of Fukaya moxibustion, writes that these points are good for neurosis, psychosis, depression, schizophrenia, dizziness, tinnitus, dystonia, and symptoms of cold such as chills, cough, runny nose, and sputum.[96]

Bamboo can be substituted for *okyu*. Note which intervertebral spaces are tender and treat. In my practice, I check every intervertebral space between T-2 and T-9, not just the five points of the Du Mai. Lay the bamboo on its side and knock gently with two fingers or a knuckle until the points release (104). If patients don't like knocking, you can roll the bamboo. Vibrating is also effective.

When focusing on a single point in this way, pay close attention to the temperature of the skin and remove the bamboo at regular intervals to avoid discomfort. The skin may become slightly red during treatment, but the tenderness at the points should release quite quickly.

---

94   Fukushima, T. (2011) *Johaibu Tokumyaku Goketsu*. Retrieved from http://www.human-world.co.jp/ahaki_world/newsitem/11/0427/110427_2_kanwa.html

95   Birch, S., & Ida, J. (1998) *Japanese Acupuncture: A Clinical Guide*. Brookline: Paradigm Publications, p. 125.

96   Fukushima, T. (2011) *Johaibu Tokumyaku Goketsu*. Retrieved from http://www.human-world.co.jp/ahaki_world/newsitem/11/0427/110427_2_kanwa.html

Always start with the most reactive point and then recheck. Frequently, when this point changes, the rest will, too. This treatment has structural benefits, and these points are always worth checking out in cases of upper back stiffness.

Insomnia

Bamboo can be used to treat insomnia. It can even be given to patients for self-help on sleepless nights.

To treat insomnia, you must bear in mind that exhausted patients need lighter treatment. Whatever you were just planning to do, reduce it by half. Dosage is discussed in detail in chapter 10, but a good rule of thumb is to do less with sleep-deprived or jetlagged patients.

Following root treatment, you can apply a very brief Bamboo Mini, focusing on the same steps as for hot flushes, but with a shorter duration:

- Release the shoulders and neck.
- Balance the upper and lower by treating the inner bladder line.
- Pul down from the head by treating the legs, especially the soles of the feet.

In addition, palpate Fukaya's anxiety points in the intervertebral spaces from T-3 to T-9. If any are tender or reactive, lay the bamboo on its side and knock gently with two fingers or a knuckle until they release.

Warm bamboo is also useful for insomnia as a self-administered home treatment, but it is essential to train patients to keep their nighttime treatments brief. Nighttime is a yin time, and Ontake is yang. While still getting the hang of Ontake treatment, I overtreated myself one night and became hugely energised, staring at the ceiling and writing notes to myself that read, "Don't moxa at night!"

In fact, moxa at night can be helpful, if kept short. If you or your patients are tossing and turning, a very brief intervention with Ontake lasting two to four minutes can be instantly helpful. If treating yourself, then tapping on the midline of the face is useful (104).

- Start just within the hairline (DU 24) and press gently with the side of the bamboo down your face, all the way to the sternal notch (REN 22). Repeat two more times.
- Press around the orbit of the eye with the lip of the bamboo (108).
- Hold the bamboo on HT 7 on both sides for a few seconds, until warm.
- Stop!

Make sure your patient is familiar with the pitfalls and dangers of using bamboo on the face, especially that protruding anatomy such as the eyeball or nose can penetrate the mouth of the bamboo and get burned.

If treating a partner, then a rapid Bamboo Mini plus legs treatment is beneficial, focusing more on the calves and feet. It is essential to keep these night treatments short and light. If you treat too long, your partner will get energised, which defeats the purpose of the exercise and may get you into trouble.

Food Poisoning and Diarrhoea

This section adapts various moxibustion approaches taught in classes by Stephen Birch and Junko Ida or presented in *Japanese Acupuncture: A Clinical Guide*[97] to treat diarrhoea using small cone moxibustion, cone moxa, and warm needling. The adaptations presented here highlight how easy it can be to import principles of treatment from other modalities into effective treatment with Ontake meridian frequency moxibustion.

In my clinical experience, diarrhoea and loose stools respond exceptionally well to bamboo. In TCM thinking, whether the problem stems from excess or deficiency, heat or cold, or if a person has had diarrhoea for a long time, you end up with spleen deficiency.[98] Knowing this and how exhausting diarrhoea can be, it is no wonder that warming the abdomen with bamboo can bring such a feeling of relief, both in acute and chronic cases.

Start with very light abdominal palpation, stroking the belly with the same lightness that you would use to stroke a nervous cat. Note signs of *kyo* and *jitsu*, observing areas of coolness, moisture, and weakness, and chart the tighter or more sensitive areas. When you have a sense of the temperature map, start warming the coldest areas very gently. When working on the abdomen, I generally use the stomach and spleen frequency for the broad strokes and kidney and Ren Mai frequencies when working on the midline.*[99]

- Tap or touch and close in a half-circle, working clockwise and using almost no pressure (132).
- When you feel the belly has relaxed somewhat, roll very lightly across the whole abdomen (132).

---

97   Birch, S., & Ida, J. (1998) *Japanese Acupuncture: A Clinical Guide.* Brookline: Paradigm Publications.

98   Maciocia, G. (1994). *The Practice of Chinese Medicine: The Treatment of Diseases with Acupuncture and Chinese Herbs.* Edinburgh: Churchill Livingstone, p. 462.

*99   This process can be viewed on YouTube (https://youtu.be/I4aBQnL2KHc), or search for Ontake Warm Bamboo Treating the Belly.

- Palpate in a circle around the navel and note any tight points. You can list them as hours of the clock, noting, for example, tightness at twelve o'clock, four o'clock, and nine o'clock. With the bamboo on its side, knock lightly at the appropriate frequency (120 or 104). Each tight point should release and feel easier on palpation. Other techniques that may help include pressing, rolling, or rocking.
- Stand or rock on the navel (104). Avoid this if the navel is convex and could protrude into the mouth of the bamboo.

These clock-around-the-navel reactions are very common in cases of acute diarrhoea and food poisoning, but for chronic diarrhoea, it is also worth palpating in a larger circle that includes both ST 25s, REN 10 to REN12, and REN 6.

- When the patient turns over, check the lower back and look for *jitsu* or *kyo* points around BL 20, 21, and BL 22 (level with T-11, T-12, and L-1). Stand, press, or roll (112).
- Touch and close on the sacrum (104).

If there has been food poisoning, you can add the very useful extra point *uranaitei*, located on the plantar surface of the foot, directly below ST 44. Locate it by bending the second toe and seeing where it makes contact with the sole (some toes won't bend, so you have to project the landing point). Hold the warm lip or side of the bamboo on the point for one to four bars (132).*[100]

Case

Male: 46. Pancreatitis.

A bit of an oil and gas industry wide boy, he had collapsed two years previously with pancreatitis. Poor diet, too much alcohol, and stress at work all contributed. He slowly rebuilt his lifestyle, making healthier choices, but when he came for acupuncture, he was troubled by stomach pain, loose, mucousy stools, and intense sacral pain whenever he ate something that disagreed with him.

The sort of patient who prefers to come for crisis management rather than for remedial or preventative treatment, he came intermittently over a couple of years whenever "the acupuncture juice ran out". He must have once been quite fit and robust, but by this time he was bony and thin. Root treatment consisted of either Manaka's pancreatitis treatments or supplementing liver and kidney channels.

---

*100 For a definition of bars, see chapter 5.

Bamboo felt very comforting and relieving when applied and rapidly released reactions on the abdomen (132, 120, or 104). Rolling on the sacrum relieved the pain (104 or 112). Bamboo Mini was very helpful, as he had lost much weight, and his skin lustre and musculature were very *kyo*.

Strangely, he found the very light needling part of Toyohari-style acupuncture slightly hard to accept, but he loved bamboo, which had an obvious cause and effect. "I don't really understand what you're doing, but when you roll that thing on my back, the pain just vanishes." His pragmatic reaction is a testament to the instant comfort of bamboo.

Constipation

Address constipation from the front and the back. As with diarrhoea, start with very light abdominal palpation, stroking the belly with the same lightness that you would use to stroke a nervous cat. Note signs of *kyo* and *jitsu*, observing areas of coolness, moisture, and weakness, and chart the tighter or more sensitive areas. When you have a picture in your mind of the coldest areas, start warming very gently with bamboo (132). Once the whole abdomen is warm, start to knock lightly on any tight points you've encountered, working around the large intestine in a clockwise direction. Once the patient is very relaxed, you can use leaning to press deeply, followed by light rolling. Leaning breaks up stagnation, and rolling spreads the qi and blood.

It is also worth palpating, rolling, and pressing along the tibia from ST36 to ST 41, ironing out any kinks and bumps along the stomach channel.

On the lower back look for *jitsu* or *kyo* points around BL 20, BL 21, and BL 22 (level with T-11, T-12, and L-1).

Eczema

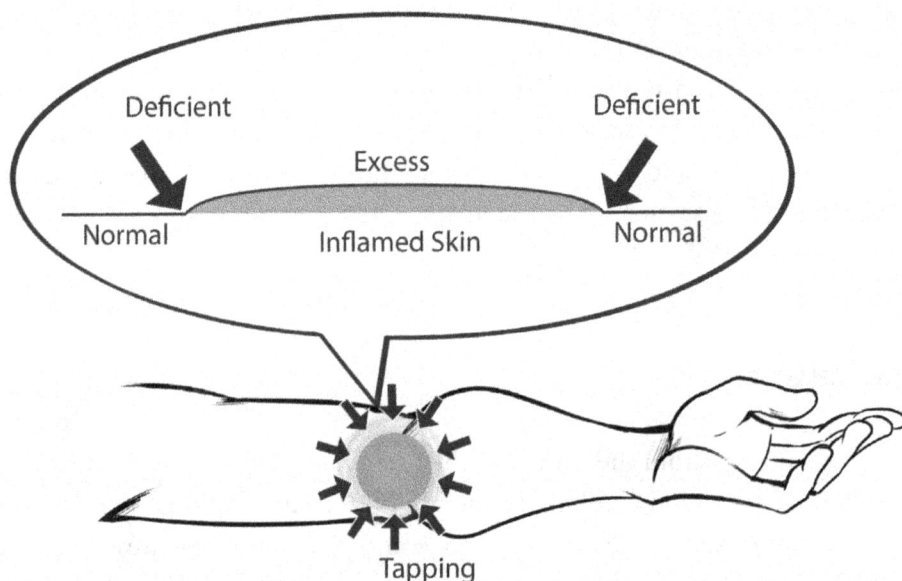

Tap around areas of inflammation, not on them.

Eczema can be seen as a local disturbance of yin and yang. The raised red area is *jitsu*, and the skin surrounding the lesion is *kyo*. In Japanese acupuncture, this theory is made practical by supplementing the qi flow on the borders of the lesion either by needling or by the application of moxa cones. Touching and closing with bamboo around the borders of a patch of eczema is a superb and efficient application of this principle. Not only is it as effective as cone moxa, but it is far quicker to apply. In the time it takes to treat one patch with moxa cones, you can treat many patches with bamboo, even if on the face or the scalp.

Supplementary points, such as LI 4, LI 11 and LI 15, may also be treated if tender. Roll or press until tenderness is reduced (108).

Cases

Female (Post-Natal): 37. Anxiety, Exhaustion, and Whole-Body Muscle Stiffness.

Root treatment was to supplement lung and spleen channels and drain the liver. Branch treatment was Bamboo Mini. She felt significantly better after the first two treatments, and on her third, she mentioned that she had eczema around her left nipple. The eczema was red and so raised she could not get a seal with her breast pump. After receiving consent, tapping lightly around the borders of the lesion

(132) stopped the itching immediately. The swelling reduced by 50 percent the same evening.

Female: 35. Atopic Dermatitis.

   Her back and abdomen were covered in patches of irritated skin. She had smaller patches on her chin and left cheek. Root treatment involved supplementing the liver and kidney channels and draining spleen excess. Bamboo was used frequently to treat the borders of the lesions on her back and abdomen. Her facial outbreak cleared up rapidly, and the lesions on her torso grew smaller every week. Sometimes, when stressed, a new patch would appear on her face, and then bamboo was used right away to stop it from getting worse. With root treatment, *okyu* (small cone moxibustion) at LI 15 and local bamboo, she made a full recovery.

Infertility

Infertility is a complicated condition that needs to be treated at the root level. As far as branch treatment with bamboo is concerned, your approach should be informed by the kind of assessment you have already made at the root level. Are the problems arising from a cold, hot, deficiency, or excess condition? If stemming from excess, is there considerable stagnation of qi, blood, and body fluids?

   As usual, palpation helps you decide how to treat. If the lustre of the abdomen is rough and deficient, touching and closing or light tapping can be used to improve the energy flow. The most straightforward use of bamboo is to warm the abdomen where it feels cold, especially the lower abdomen.

   Moreover, bamboo can be helpful in conditions of stagnation and accumulation and can be applied to the leg on the spleen and liver channel, as well as on the abdomen. If there are tight points around the ASIS, tap lightly at 132 beats per minute until they release.

   On the back, fertility issues often reflect with deficiency or stagnation signs over the sacrum. Deficiency manifests with cold or puffy skin, while excess signs may show with tightness, swelling and pressure pain. There may also be tight, swollen areas on the bladder channel around BL 23.

   Japanese sources recommend gentle "sensing warmth" direct moxibustion with large cones over sacral manifestations of deficiency. Bamboo is an efficient and quick way to apply this warming heat, and if applied more vigorously at the bladder or Du Mai frequencies, it can also be used to unblock stagnation in the area.

Inducing Labour

This should be combined with other methods but is a useful adjunctive therapy. In Chinese acupuncture, LI 4, GB 21, SP 6, and sometimes LIV 3 are stimulated strongly.[101] In Japanese acupuncture, prolonged small cone moxibustion on SP-6 is recommended.

Any patient who is coming for labour induction can usually be classified as anxious, because most doctors give patients a deadline, and going beyond that deadline means treatment involves chemical labour induction, or worse. It is a sad observation, particularly here in Malaysia, that many doctors regard pregnancy as a pathology to be managed rather than a natural process. On so many occasions, the subliminal message is "You're not pregnant—you're in danger!", whereas the mother's reality is actually, "I'm not sick—I'm pregnant!"

Sometimes, chemical induction is proposed purely for administrative reasons, not medical reasons. Occasionally, patients seek early induction in week thirty-eight for other reasons; for example, if the baby has already grown so big that they are worried about the labour at forty or forty-one weeks.

Whatever the reason, most patients feel anxious and under pressure—quite often tired and exhausted as well. As we have already seen, there is something wonderfully relaxing about bamboo treatment, and it therefore should be included during acupuncture for labour induction procedures, both to calm the mind and to open up the lower back and pelvis.

- With the patient sitting, roll, press, or release GB 21 if tight (120).
- Press either side of the bladder channel from the upper back to the lumbar region (112).
- Roll the sacrum at 104 beats per minute and 112 beats per minute.
- Tap or press along the iliac crest on both sides from PSIS to ASIS (120).
- Tap and press lightly in the inguinal groove at 132 beats per minute.

It may be helpful to bring in relevant aspects of Bamboo Max on the arms and legs. Take your time. This should be very relaxing, as this kind of patient is inherently anxious about the event to come. Bamboo treatment should induce deep feelings of warmth, letting go, and opening in the lower abdomen. Together with regular treatment, this should help trigger labour.

It is worth adding here that the pain relief protocols in the next chapter work magically for all the aches, pains, and discomforts of pregnancy (see the included cases).

---

101   Flaws, B., (1983). *The Path of Pregnancy: Classical Chinese Medical Perspectives on Conception, Pregnancy, Delivery, and Postpartum Care.* Brookline: Paradigm Publications.

Children

Children love bamboo treatments. They like the clicking of the metronome, the smell of moxa, and the comforting warmth. It can be a fun game to let them blow on the ash in the bamboo until it glows, but be careful not to let them too close, in case they blow too hard and ash flies into their eyes. Treatment time needs to be considerably shorter for children, from two or three minutes to just a few seconds.

As usual, bamboo can be used as an adjunctive treatment to the essential root treatment. For example, for colic in babies, just a few seconds of rolling on the abdomen at 132 beats per minute or unaccompanied can be very beneficial. For bedwetting in older children, rolling on the lumbar area (112) and the lower Ren and kidney points (104 or 120) has proved very helpful. In babies and infants, digestion is often at the root of all kinds of manifestations. Many conditions, even insomnia and night terrors respond to just a few seconds of rolling or touching and closing on the abdomen at 132 beats per minute.

Case

Female: 4 Months. Sinus Trouble.

Her mother was concerned that there was a sinus problem. The baby's nose would get blocked at feeding time, and she kept rejecting her mother's breast. It was as if she couldn't breathe, and she would get red in the face and cry. If her mother cleaned her nose, things got easier. The baby was examined by two different paediatricians, but they essentially said there was nothing wrong with her.

She had a calm temperament (except at feeding time), was gaining weight, and slept well.

On the first session, root treatment focused on treating the spleen with a *teishin* (a blunt silver probe) at SP-3, and Shonishin massage with an *enshin* (a rounded silver stroking tool) on the channels. Branch treatment included touching and closing with Ontake on the tummy, without a metronome, for ten seconds. We taught the mother the Shonishin routine and how to apply Ontake on the tummy and sent her home with an *enshin*, bamboo, and moxa.

After the first treatment, there was a significant improvement. After the second week, the mother described her as a different child, with no more fuss or drama at mealtimes.

Loading, lighting, and rolling with Ontake can be taught to mothers very quickly. A concern that has been raised with this idea is that the mother might fail to compress the moxa enough and allow hot ash to fall on her little patient, but this concern goes against basic maternal instincts. Moreover, you can teach mothers to apply the bamboo on its side, making it harder for the ash to fall out. You can also instruct them to apply Ontake through clothing as an extra level of precaution.

Stroke

It seems valuable to close this chapter with an extended case study of a man treated for stroke with a combination of acupuncture, moxibustion, and Ontake. Many of the bamboo treatments were given at the branch level, and some of the treatments served as precedents for the whole-body treatments described earlier. The case was serious and complicated, and demonstrates the power and adaptability of Ontake to aid recovery.

Male: 46. Embolic Stroke

"Richard" was an expat living in Kuala Lumpur and working in the hospitality industry. He gave up smoking with the help of acupuncture in 2009 and then stopped coming for treatment. In the year that followed, he started to overeat, and his cholesterol and blood pressure went up. Eventually, he had an embolic stroke while swimming. He was treated in the hospital for three weeks, and just a week after discharge, he came for acupuncture. This is one of the double-edged aspects of treating smokers. Weight gain is commonplace after stopping smoking, but most patients seldom continue treatment after stopping smoking.

On his first visit, Richard was in a wheelchair. He could barely move his right arm and leg, and his face and eye were also slightly affected. Both his right hand and foot were ice cold. His pulse was thin but excess, deep, and slightly rapid. With assistance, he was able to hobble and lurch from his wheelchair to the treatment table, but he was very unstable.

Root treatment was to supplement the lung and drain liver excess. Branch treatment was *kikei* on the large intestine and stomach channels. This method involved placing a copper pellet on LI 4 and a zinc pellet on ST 43, using the differing electrovalence of the two metals to create a microvoltage between the two points, with the skin as a conductor.

Bamboo was applied on all the yang channels of the arm and leg from hand to shoulder and hip to foot, tapping at the appropriate channel frequencies. His hand immediately grew hot, and his foot grew warm.

Four days later, he returned with greater movement and control in his leg. His physiotherapist had immediately noticed the improvement. His hand had remained warm, ever since the first treatment, and his foot was cool, not icy. The pulse was now much softer. Root treatment was the same.

Branch treatment continued without *kikei*, just with bamboo. Three days later, he moved much more confidently from wheelchair to table. His movements were stronger, and he was able to move his arm from the shoulder. His doctors noticed some spasticity in his fingers and wanted to inject with Botox. Root treatment was the same, but a variation of *kikei* was applied. The spasticity was very mild—surely not reason for Botox injections—and it was relieved immediately with the application of the copper. *Shiraku* (bloodletting) was applied at the *jing*-well points of pericardium and lung channels (three drops).

Bamboo was applied at the yin channel frequencies (176 and 126) on the arm and to the stomach, spleen, gall bladder, and kidney channels on the leg. After applying the bamboo on his arm, he was—for the first time—able to move his index finger. Despite this improvement, he was injected with Botox the next day.

On his fourth treatment, he requested treatment for his eyesight. Previously, the left had been his good eye, but since his stroke, it was not tracking well. He was contemplating corrective eye surgery for his right eye, which was short-sighted but tracking normally. On inspection, his right eye moved normally, but his left eye moved from side to side and was unable to follow my moving finger.

Treatment involved MSA, using ion-pumping cords connecting the upper and lower meeting points of the yin and yang channels (NIP 1).[102] Ontake was applied on his arm, leg, and around the eye (108). On his next visit, he reported that after two hours, there was a sudden and dramatic shift in his visual tracking and acuity. On inspection, it was clear that there had been a remarkable improvement in tracking and coordination.

On his sixth treatment, Richard mentioned that a large area from under his armpit to his pelvis was still numb (mostly the spleen channel). His thumb was a little stiff, and his hand was colder than usual. Toyohari was selected for root treatment this time.

Branch treatment included rolling bamboo from LU 1 to LU 11 (126), LI 1 to LI 20 (108), ST 1 to ST 44 (132), and SP 1 to SP 21 (132). Some readers will recognise this sequence as the first four-channel set of the Chinese Clock: lung, large intestine, stomach, and spleen (for more information about four-channel sets, see chapter 11).

Treatment was very brisk, taking only five minutes to complete the whole four-channel circuit. By the end of this, he had a feeling of warmth deep inside both his

---

102 Matsumoto, K., & Birch S. (1988). *Hara Diagnosis: Reflections on the Sea*, Brookline: Paradigm Publications, pp. 389–393.

arm and leg and hugely increased sensation all over the previously numb area. His thumb lost all its spasticity.

Richard continued treatment for a year, gradually reducing his frequency of treatment. He made rapid progress, quickly discarding the wheelchair, then his crutches, and then the walking stick. The recovery of his arm was somewhat slower, especially for simple tasks like grasping and turning a door handle, but his overall recovery was excellent. At the end of the year, he moved to another country, and I never got to see the final outcome.

Looking back, Richard was an extraordinary patient, blessed with an uncompromising and driving will to recover. Much of his rapid recovery was due to this. Nevertheless, both he and I felt that, from day one, Ontake was a significant component of his rehabilitation success story.

Summary

On the face of it, this chapter is about ways to treat symptoms with Ontake, but underlying each routine is a reliance on palpation and the identification of abnormal tissues, such as tenderness, coolness, or crunchy crystals.

Branch treatment is usually added at the end of a treatment, when the patient's energy is more ordered and can be integrated into any system. Sometimes it is applied first, or concurrently.

How many symptoms should we treat in one session and how much treatment should we give? The next chapter considers how much is enough.

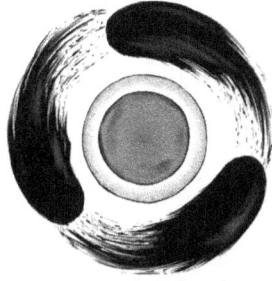

CHAPTER 10

DOSAGE AND THE GOLDILOCKS ZONE

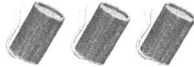

Defining, anticipating, and dealing with overtreatment and how to recognise each person's unique limits for treatment.

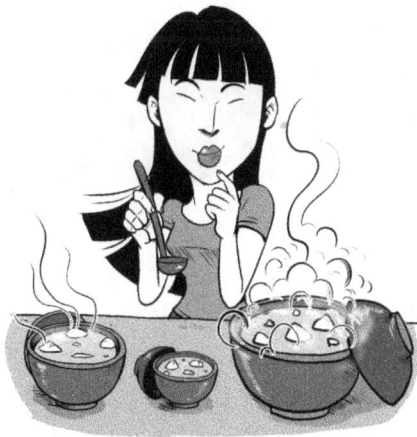

"This porridge is too hot!" Goldilocks exclaimed. She clambered down off the big chair and moved to the next place at the table. Next, she tasted the porridge in the second bowl.

"This porridge is too cold!" she said. Again, she moved chairs and sampled the porridge in the third bowl.

This time the porridge was neither too hot nor too cold.

"Mmmm, this porridge is just right," she said with glee, and she ate it all, down to the very last drop!

In Robert Southey's fairy tale *Goldilocks and the Three Bears*, first published in 1837, a rather intrusive little girl enters uninvited into the house of three variously sized bears. Fortunately, they are not at home, so she shamelessly sets about sampling their breakfast, sitting on their kitchen furniture and climbing into their beds. This fastidious little girl judges the porridge to be too hot, too cold, or just right; the chairs are too big, too small, or just right; and their beds are too hard, too soft, or just right.

The term "Goldilocks Zone" means the range of values that is neither too high nor too low but is just right for a given function. It has even found its way into cosmology to describe that distance from a star that is neither too hot nor too cold for carbon-based life like us to exist.

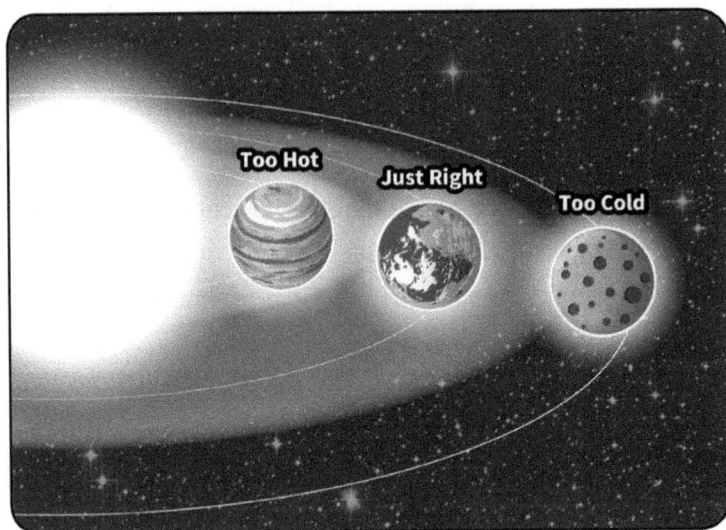

The Goldilocks Zone in the solar system.

What is the Goldilocks Zone for treatment with acupuncture and moxibustion? When is a treatment too much, when is it not enough, and when is it just right?

This chapter reiterates ideas about dosage first presented by Dr Manaka and disseminated by Stephen Birch, as well as thinking and practice from instructors in the Toyohari Association in Japan. Although this book is about Ontake, the concepts that inform this chapter can be used for the planning and execution of all treatments, no matter your style of acupuncture or bodywork.

Maximum Benefit with Minimal Intervention

Continuous effort should be made to perform therapy using the minimum number of acupuncture points possible ... although the amount of stimulation may be increased when the need arises, care must be taken not to exceed the individual's limit beyond which unnecessary side effects arise.

—Manaka, Itaya, and Birch[103]

The idea that there is a limit to treatment "beyond which unnecessary side effects arise" is crucial to understanding dosage in acupuncture. In Western medicine, drug dosage is related to many criteria, age and body weight being most important. For example, a doctor may prescribe a child a quarter of an aspirin pill, and an adult two whole pills. An elderly or frail patient may need only one. Patients can, therefore, be divided into two groups: sensitive and robust.

If these two categories sound familiar, it is because we have already encountered their Japanese equivalents when discussing *kyo* and *jitsu*. Beyond the meaning of "excess" that we have previously discussed in earlier chapters, *jitsu* has another meaning relating to health: "robustness" or "strength". Someone who is *jitsu* can be said to be in "rude good health", strong and full of life. In clinical practice, this means that robust patients can tolerate acupuncture much better than sensitive patients. Thus, it is essential for us to do two things:

- Identify patients as either robust or sensitive, and treat them differently.
- Recognise the signs, both good and bad, that show we have given sufficient treatment.

Advantages of a Gradualist Clinical Approach

A few years ago, an elderly patient of mine borrowed her neighbour's car while hers was being repaired. Her own car was a very antiquated and sedate automatic, a real-life example of the second-hand car advert featuring "one careful lady owner". Her neighbour's car, also automatic, was more powerful and highly tuned. Within thirty seconds of starting the engine, she had accelerated through her garden gate, just managing to brake outside her living room patio doors. She ended up with a few

---

103   Manaka, Y., Itaya, K., & Birch, S. (1995). *Chasing the Dragon's Tail: The Theory and Practice of Acupuncture in the Work of Yoshio Manaka*. Brookline: Paradigm Publications, p. 116.

bruises, a sprained wrist (which responded well to Ontake), and some injured pride (which did not).

Slow cars and fast cars offer the same outcome: they both get you to where you want to go. Similarly, both low-stimulation and strong-stimulation methods aim to improve your patients' energy. One crucial difference is that slow cars and low-stimulation methods give you much more control over the journey. Without that control, you may overshoot badly, especially if you are treating sensitive patients.

"Overtreatment" can have many adverse consequences, including fatigue, nausea, light-headedness, or aggravated symptoms. The late Mr Takai, former President of the Toyohari Association of Japan, stated simply that he believed 90 percent of adverse reactions in his clinic over the forty years were due to overtreatment.[104] Dr Manaka first explained this concept in *Chasing the Dragon's Tail.*

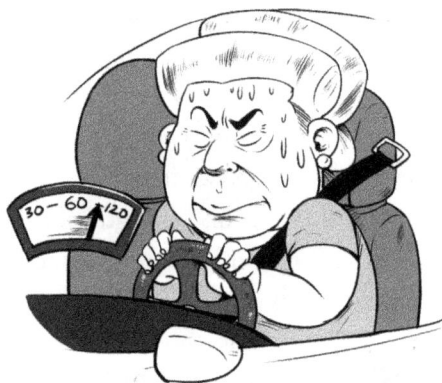

Fast cars can overshoot the destination.

Dr Manaka's Graph of Stimulus and Reaction

This graph shows Manaka's model for contrasting strong and mild methods of treatment.[105] There are three horizontal bands representing insufficient, adequate, and excessive dosages of treatment. An insufficient dose will not cause a curative effect. Too much will cause adverse reactions. Our ideal treatment dosage should fall in the Goldilocks Zone: not too much, not too little—but just right.

---

104   Clinic visit during Toyohari Summer School. (2000). Tokyo.

105   Manaka, Y., Itaya, K., & Birch, S. (1995). *Chasing the Dragon's Tail: The Theory and Practice of Acupuncture in the Work of Yoshio Manaka.* Brookline: Paradigm Publications, p. 119.

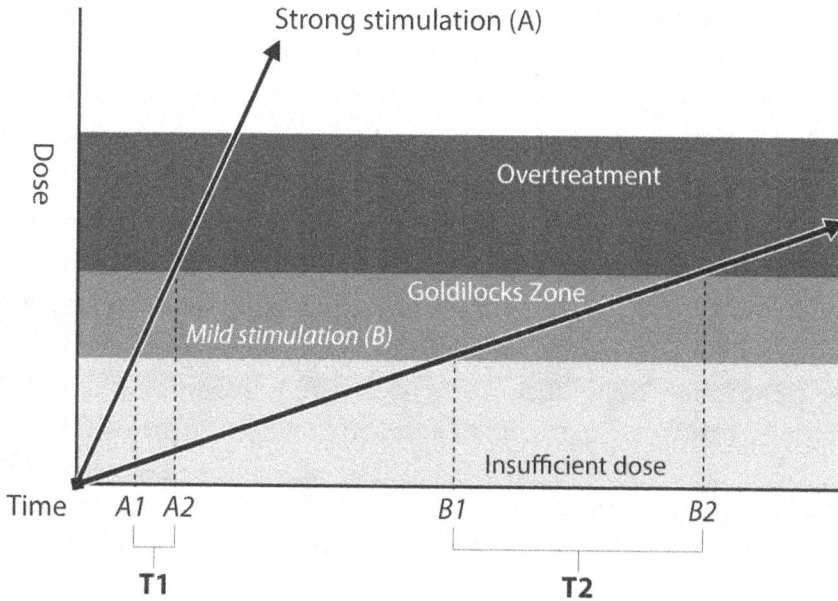

The Goldilocks Zone for the average patient.

Treatment A, using strong physical stimulation, can arrive at the correct dosage quickly, but, like the neighbour's powerful car, can easily overshoot, causing adverse reactions. If we measure from the time that the dosage reaches the Goldilocks Zone (A1) to the time it exceeds it (A2), we can see the time is quite short (T1).

Treatment B, using low-intensity stimuli, uses a series of carefully monitored low dose interventions to reach an effective level of stimulation. In this instance, if we measure from the same two points, B1 and B2, we can see that there is much more time to monitor the effects of the treatment effects (T2) and stop at the right time. There is less chance of overtreating the patient.

Both in Toyohari and MSA, treatment consists of incremental steps. Each step is monitored for its effect, with feedback mechanisms specific to the method used. Both styles have researched and developed devices and techniques that apply small or minute stimuli to the meridian system.

This approach is taken for all patients, but particular care should be taken for sensitive patients, which includes the elderly, the very young, and anyone who might react strongly to standard treatment.

The benefits of this gradualist, gentle approach to treatment include:
- Greater control over therapeutic effects
- Increased time to assess and regulate treatment
- A reduction in adverse reactions from incorrect treatment and overtreatment
- Increased patient comfort and relaxation from low-stimulation techniques

Identifying Sensitive Patients

As we have established, some patients are more sensitive than others. To plan our dosage and treatment, we need to identify this kind of person right away. Sometimes we can do this simply from their appearance: they look weak, skinny or tired.

Age is also a key factor. We must assume that the very young and the very old are more sensitive. Of course, we will encounter very robust elderly patients from time to time, but as a general rule, it is safe to assume that the older they are, the more sensitive they will be. If it seems obvious that a ninety-nine-year-old with back pain should be treated more gently than a thirty-year-old, it is worth noting that by the same principle, a sixty-year-old should be treated more gently than a fifty-year-old. Likewise, a weak or tired-looking fifty-year-old should be treated more gently than a healthy-looking patient of the same age.

Age is at the top of the list as an indicator for sensitivity, although there are many other signs that might warn you that certain patients are more sensitive than others:

- Age: they are very young or very old.
- They have been ill for a long time.
- They are literally sensitive: They "feel" things. They can "sense" things. They receive "guidance". Some spiritual people are very sensitive and require minimal treatment.
- They do a lot of work on themselves and their own qi. This includes "therapy junkies" and people constantly engaged in yoga, spa treatments, personal growth work, and counselling.
- They are artistic, creative, or reflective.
- They have some emotional trauma (recent or old). If they start crying during the pre-treatment chat, it is a clear indication to do a light treatment.
- They talk a lot, and it's hard to get them to relax.

What Is a Sensitive Patient?

Mr Nakada, the former President of the Toyohari Association, reported that volubility is a very obvious indicator of sensitivity. In a lecture on dosage, he said unequivocally, "If a patient talks a lot, use fewer needles!"[106]

Why would this be? We all have had patients who talk a lot; sometimes, it is difficult to obtain relevant information from them, even though they use so many words. Sometimes they do not hear our questions correctly and spend a long time

---

106 Toyohari Summer School. (2010). Tokyo.

answering something else, or they get emotionally re-stimulated to talk about something irrelevant or provide irrelevant detail.

Of course, this is a pathology in itself. For someone to interact and talk in this way, there must be, in very basic terms, an imbalance of yin and yang. The yin is not anchoring the yang. This is a volatile state and must, therefore, be treated with particular caution. At its worst, this is a psychotic state. Reducing the dosage is the first step to successful treatment.

We can use the example of volubility to try and understand all the above conditions that lead to sensitivity. At first, the list above may seem strange. Why should we put people with past trauma in the same treatment category as those who invest in their health by doing a lot of Tai Chi or yoga? Surely, one group is traumatised and the other is healthy?

If we consider these two groups, it is apparent that there is some crossover between them; many people with past trauma are led to work on themselves. However, whether people do meditation, have a chronic disease, or talk a lot, what they have in common is an energy system that is sensitive to nudges, either because it is very finely tuned or somewhat out of balance.

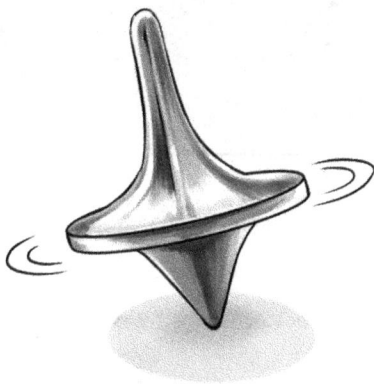

This spinning top is sensitive to nudges.

One way of picturing this is to imagine a child's spinning top. When it is spinning, it should be upright, but for some reason, it may be leaning to one side. This is a finely tuned, sensitive person. To push it to the upright position requires the gentlest of nudges. If you push too far, it will tip the other way, and your patient will feel worse after treatment. Another spinning top might be wobbling eccentrically. Once again, small nudges are required to get it back up to speed. A big nudge may destabilise it completely. Overtreatment can, therefore, be seen as pushing an individual too forcefully, overshooting Goldilocks Zone of healing and passing into a new zone of counter-reaction.

The Goldilocks Zone for Sensitive Patients

Using Manaka's model of treatment, we can see in the diagram below that sensitive patients present quite differently. The Goldilocks Zone changes in two crucial ways.

First of all, it is lower on the y-axis (vertical) than that of a normal, robust patient. Less treatment is needed to achieve an adequate dose. Secondly, it is narrower on the y-axis than a robust patient's zone. This means that, just like my elderly patient in the powerful car, it is now even easier to give too much stimulation and to overshoot in a shorter space of time (T1).

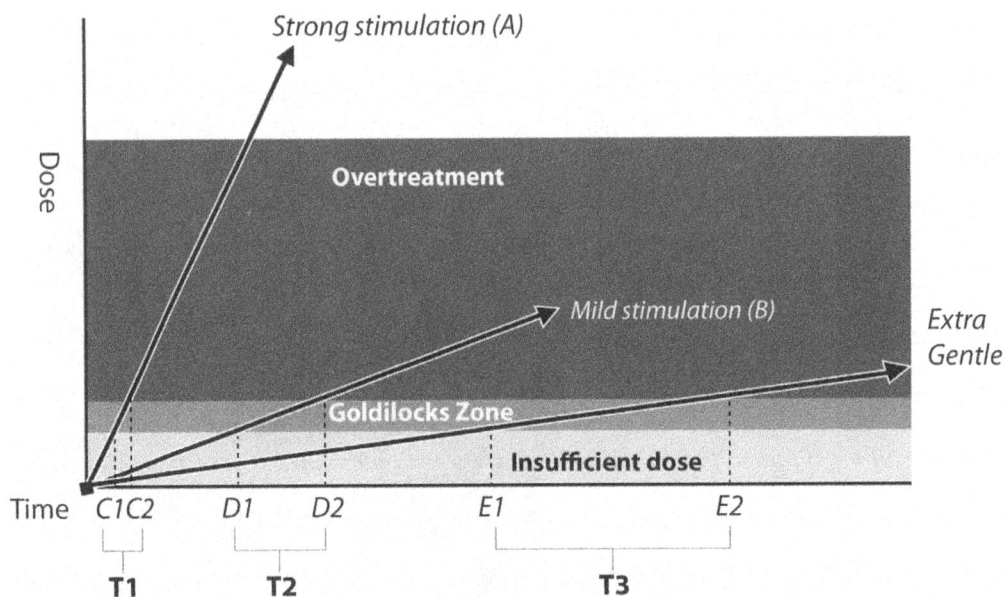

The Goldilocks Zone for a sensitive patient.

Even with normal gentle treatment, T2 is shorter. Thus, with this kind of sensitive or hyper-sensitive patient, it makes sense to use an even gentler gradient of treatment, meaning that you should apply especially mild methods of stimulation (T3).

Feedback Mechanisms and Warning Signs

Most acupuncturists use a variety of feedback mechanisms to assess the effectiveness of their treatment. These include:

- Improvements in pulse quality
- Relief of pressure pain on treatment points and the *hara*
- Improvements in the mobility of affected joints
- Improvements in skin lustre

- Symptom relief
- Patient feedback and participation

These same feedback mechanisms can also be used as indicators of a treatment going from the Goldilocks Zone to overtreatment.

Warning signs include:

- Pulse quality deteriorates, notably becoming weaker, more floating and rapid
- Previously relaxed areas start to tighten up again, including treatment areas, treatment points, and the *hara*
- The skin starts to get cold or moist
- Whole-body sweating
- The patient's state changes from relaxed to restless (you will note that after a long period of not moving, their head starts to turn from side to side)
- Complaints of feeling faint, weak, or dizzy
- Needle shock, as defined in Chinese acupuncture

Modifying Dosage for Elderly or Sensitive Patients

As we can see from Manaka's model of treatment, the simplest method to reduce the dosage of treatment is to reduce the treatment duration. Secondly, we can select lighter techniques. For example, we can use shallower needling, finer needles, and fewer points.

In terms of moxibustion, we can use less heat and fewer cones, applying larger warming cones rather than small, hot ones. Ontake can be applied in the gentlest way with sensitive patients, with the option of omitting the metronome and going unaccompanied.

Finally, it is better to work more on *kyo* than *jitsu*, supplementing rather than draining. In these cases, it is better to use gentler Ontake techniques: touching and closing, light rolling and tapping.

Dealing with Overtreatment in the Clinic

If you note any of the signs above and believe you may have done too much, you should remove the needles, exactly as you would for needle shock.

If the patient feels very faint, let them lie with their knees up to bring blood to the head. Apply heat with unaccompanied Ontake, a moxa stick, or cone moxa at DU 14. In the Toyohari Association, DU 14 is the primary point for recovery from wrong treatment or overtreatment, but if the patient is supine, you can treat REN 4. If the knees are bent, then REN 4 is trickier to access, so select ST 36 instead.

After-Effects of Overtreatment

Sometimes overtreatment can wrongly be interpreted by practitioners and patients as a favourable healing crisis, often described by forgiving patients with phrases such as, "I must be getting rid of toxins". "No pain, no gain", and "Things have to get worse before they get better".

Sometimes patients have a genuine healing crisis following treatment, a worsening of symptoms that precedes recovery. In Japanese, this is called *mengen*. In the Toyohari Association, *mengen* is defined as fatigue or aggravation of symptoms following treatment that lasts no more than twenty-four hours.

If the patient feels bad for longer than this, you can assume that your treatment exceeded "the individual's limit beyond which unnecessary side effects arise".[107] Examples of this include:
- Fatigue which lasts more than twenty-four hours
- Worsening symptoms
- New symptoms[108]
- Poor sleep

Feeling tired after treatment is not bad at all. If it lasts more than twenty-four hours, it can be considered overtreatment. Poor sleep after treatment is not unusual, and if your patient mentions this at the next session, this is a significant and easy-to-interpret cue to moderate the dosage.

Case

Female: 65. Exhaustion and Hot Flushes.

This sixty-five-year-old grandmother was visiting Malaysia to see her new grandson. She had been feeling exhausted for several years. She also had many hot flushes, especially at night. Her first session was with MSA, using an ion-pumping treatment often prescribed for fatigue arising from a kidney weakness and *okyu* (small

---

107   Manaka, Y., Itaya, K., & Birch, S. (1995). *Chasing the Dragon's Tail: The Theory and Practice of Acupuncture in the Work of Yoshio Manaka.* Brookline: Paradigm Publications, p. 116.

108   Yanagishita, T. (2010). Toyohari Summer School. Tokyo.

cone moxibustion) at LI 10, REN 12, and ST 36 (three cones). Ontake was given on the back.

She returned the following week, saying that she had felt completely wiped out for two days and had been sleeping very long hours. The first night, her hot flushes were worse than ever. Following these two lousy nights, her energy picked up, and her flushes were much reduced.

Clearly, this was overtreatment. I had overestimated how much treatment she could take. Nevertheless, the treatment was on the right track, as she was feeling better. For the next treatment, the dosage was much reduced. The ion-pumping time was halved, *okyu* was repeated with one cone on each point, and the Ontake time was reduced by 75%.

If a master practitioner such as Mr Takai can admit that that most of the adverse reactions in his practice were due to overtreatment, we can forgive ourselves if we get it wrong on the first session and maybe even the second. But the reaction to the early sessions must be used to calibrate future treatments. Getting it wrong routinely is less forgivable. These days, I scrawl a big red *S* on the top page of sensitive patients' notes, so that even if they come back years later, I am still reminded to treat them with special care.

Introducing the Jitsometer

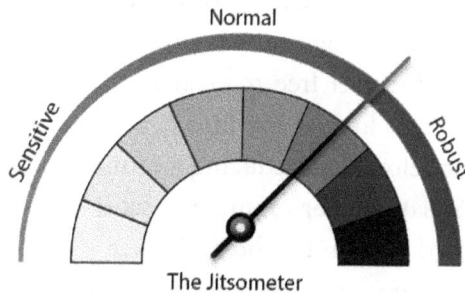

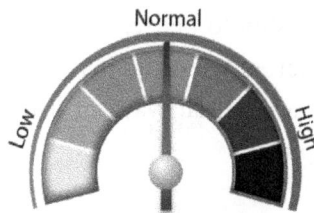

Normal

Sensitive

Robust

The Jitsometer

Normal

Low

High

The Dosimeter

Dialling it down with the jitsometer.

The "jitsometer" is a thought experiment that you can perform before you start treatment. If the word *jitsu* can be used to describe the strength and robustness of a patient's energy system, then the jitsometer is a mental way of viewing that strength. If the dial is zero on the left, five in the middle, and ten on the right—then the further to the right that the needle is on the dial, the more robust the patient is. The further to the left the needle is on the dial, the more sensitive the patient is and the less treatment you should give.

When teaching, I usually use the Kozato method, a group consensus model for practice and learning from Toyohari. One practitioner becomes the model patient, and a few others plan and carry out the treatment together. When teaching this idea, I have found it remarkable how, in group practice, there is widespread agreement by the treating group about the model patient's jitsometer score. This suggests that this is an intuitive, common-sense process. Once you have the concept of dosage and the Goldilocks Zone in your head, it is relatively easy to place people on a continuum.

The Dosimeter

The next tool is the "dosimeter", another mental needle gauge in a direct relationship to the jitsometer. In science, a dosimeter is a device used to measure exposure to doses of radiation. In this context, we will use it to refer to an internalised dial that points to the amount of stimulation with acupuncture and moxibustion you should give to your patient. If someone scores high on the jitsometer, you can set your dosimeter to one point below that and feel free to treat root and branch with any method you see fit. If someone scores low on the jitsometer, you must adjust the dosimeter downwards to one point below that, reducing treatment time, focusing more on the root and using less stimulation. For example, a score of five on the jitsometer will enable a treatment strength of four on the dosimeter,

As a rule of thumb, many patients in your practice will be somewhere around the four to six position on your dial and can be treated with a dosage of three to five. But it is worth noting that patients who score below two on the jitsometer can be classified as hypersensitive and should be treated with great care.

Of course, these are not actual scientific instruments but intuitive impressions. Nevertheless, I have found these visual ways of learning, practising, and teaching these concepts to be very helpful.

Usual and Unusual: Exceptional Circumstances

As we have seen, we can use a jitsometer in our mind's eye to classify most of our patients into three groups:

- Robust (7–10)
- Normal (4–6)
- Sensitive (0–3)

What is important to understand is that these energy states are changing all the time. If a patient comes to see you who is usually a robust seven on the jitsometer but tells you tearfully that his wife just left him, it absolutely makes sense to downgrade his rating immediately. The same thinking goes for a normal patient who is jetlagged: your mental jitsometer and dosimeters should dial down. Thus, we can add a fourth category: *unusually* sensitive patients. With this addition, we have patients who are:

- Usually robust
- Usually normal
- Usually sensitive
- Unusually sensitive

This fourth category means that those people who are usually in one place on the sensitivity spectrum may, on a given day, be less robust and more sensitive than usual. The reason may be a recent emotional trauma, lack of sleep, jet lag, recovery from illness, or a prolonged period of overwork or stress. This principle also applies to your sensitive patients. On some days, they may become hypersensitive, and this unusual situation will test your skill to the utmost to arrive at a meaningful dose of treatment without sending them over the edge.

Thus, you should never take your patients' sensitivity for granted. Always consult your jitsometer before treatment and adjust your dosimeter accordingly.

Insensitive Patients

There is one final type of patient to consider when thinking about dosage, suggested by Australian acupuncture trainer Paul Movsessian. These are patients with reduced sensitivity, and not in a good way.[109] These patients are not *jitsu* with vitality but because they have chronic blood stasis. Patients with blood stasis are usually more challenging to treat. Typical indicators of blood stasis include medical histories with

---

109 Movsessian, P. (2017). Sensitive Patients. *Keiraku Chiryo – International Toyohari News, 11*, p. 8.

multiple surgeries, elderly patients with liver channel pathologies or high blood pressure, and stubborn conditions such as psoriasis. People who tend to fall into this category are manual labourers, outdoor labourers, fruit pickers, people with excessive exposure to the sun (think of a typical farmer or fisherman), and extreme athletes. In these cases, the Goldilocks Zone may be the opposite of sensitive patients'. It may be that their threshold for effective treatment is higher.

To treat this kind of patient, you need to work in a very different way than with sensitive patients. Not only should you consider longer needle retention with more points, moxibustion techniques involving more moxa cones, and longer Ontake sessions, but you should also consider stronger methods such as *tonnetsukyu* (burning the moxa all the way down) or *shiraku* (bloodletting).

Cases

Female: 55. Breast Cancer Survivor.

This woman first had breast cancer in 2013 in her left breast. She came in for acupuncture in 2014, just weeks before she was diagnosed with triple-negative cancer in her right breast. She also had gluten intolerances and a long history of eye surgeries for retinal and macular detachment. She had supportive acupuncture in 2014 while undergoing chemotherapy and came back in 2017 for help with her vision (flashing lights and zigzag lines in her left eye), intense joint pain, and poor sleep. Typically treated with Toyohari as a liver *sho* (this means simply that the liver channel was "the weakest link"), it took two sessions to calibrate treatment to her level of sensitivity, scoring a three on the jitsometer. Signs of overtreatment included feeling super-relaxed during the session and then being unable to sleep at night.

Root treatment was with the thinnest silver needles in the clinic (number one silver needles) and touch-needling with minimal stimulation. Ontake was used primarily for pain relief, working on the normal mirror on the feet to treat her joint pains on the wrist. Moxa was with large cones, burning only the top third, removing it before she could feel any warmth, or low numbers of *okyu* (small cone moxibustion).

Over six months, all her symptoms reduced considerably. Her joint pain disappeared, and she slept well, with a significant reduction in the flashing lights.

Recently, her ninety-year-old mother visited Malaysia, and this triggered some emotional lability. She arrived in the session tearful and full of resentment. This meant that she became even more sensitive to treatment than before, now scoring a one on the jitsometer. In Toyohari, symptoms can be treated with *kikei*, which involves placing copper and zinc buttons on the master and coupled points of the

Eight Extras. This exploits the differing electrovalence of the two metals, creating a microvoltage between the two points, with the skin as a conductor.

In this patient's case, merely taping the copper button on a single acupuncture point triggered nausea. After testing several points with the same intense reaction, the procedure was abandoned. Root treatment was given with *sesshokushin* (touch needling) with a blunt gold *teishin* instead of a needle, with the bare minimum of stimulation, and a single platform moxa cone was burned on SP 1. Treatment finished with a Bamboo Mini plus legs, lasting about thirty seconds.

She returned the following week looking very chipper and with a swish in her step. This improvement likely was not due to my finely attuned acupuncture treatment but her mother's departure two days before. We upgraded her jitsometer rating to two and continue to treat her very lightly indeed.

How to Moderate Dosage with Ontake

As we have seen from Manaka's graphical representations of dosage, one of the key ways we can reduce the dosage is by making the duration of treatment shorter. This rule applies to any modality or method, be it electro-acupuncture, needling, moxibustion, cupping, or Ontake.

Ontake's effects have three main components:
- Technique (tapping, rolling, etc.)
- Moxibustion
- Frequency

Techniques

Reducing dosage by moderating the techniques can be done in three ways:
1. Technique selection
2. Reducing the strength of application
3. Reducing the duration of application

For example, some techniques feel stronger than others. Knocking and super-knocking are relatively forceful, sending a stronger signal to the body than touching and closing, or standing. Thus, to moderate the dosage, simply choose a lighter technique.

When you apply the technique, apply it with less force. For example, when rolling, roll lightly with the bamboo at your fingertips, not your palm. Tap or knock on the beat, not in double time. Use less force to tap.

Tap or roll briefly, then monitor the patient's reaction on the pulse before tapping more.

Moxibustion

It is my opinion that moxibustion provides the single most important component of Ontake treatment. Without moxibustion, Ontake becomes more on a par with Manaka's wooden needle and hammer, with which he said it was almost impossible to overtreat.[110] It absolutely is possible to overtreat with Ontake, as I saw once when teaching in Thailand. Bamboo Max should last a maximum of twenty-five minutes, but in this class, my instructions were poorly understood, and one who had been treated for more than forty minutes, went into a very uncomfortable needle shock–like reaction, feeling cold, clammy, and faint. Since then, when teaching Ontake, I designate some practice sessions as "compulsory cold practice", meaning we do not light the Ontake. Students can experiment and become familiar with the techniques without the risk of overtreatment.

Moxibustion has many different and various effects on its own. The most obvious one is the warmth of the bamboo when in contact with the skin, but there are other effects to consider, such as the infrared frequency of the burning moxa and the smell of the smoke. There may also be pharmacological effects stemming from the smoke inhalation or smoke contacting the skin.

Thus, applying Ontake without moxa is the most dramatic way to reduce the dose, a useful step to take when teaching and learning Ontake but perhaps too limiting if applied during treatment. Pragmatically, we can reduce the heat of the Ontake by using a piece of bamboo with thicker skin, by burning less moxa in the tube, or by using rapid strokes that limit contact with the skin.

Frequencies

Once again, we have to consider that applying Ontake with a metronome has effects on more than one level. Of course, there is the signature rhythmic application of heat that defines meridian frequency moxibustion. This is perceived through the skin and soft tissue, but we can also consider that the body receives the sound of the metronome frequency through the ear. As we have seen, the sound is quite

---

110   Manaka, Y., Itaya, K., & Birch, S. (1995). *Chasing the Dragon's Tail: The Theory and Practice of Acupuncture in the Work of Yoshio Manaka*. Brookline: Paradigm Publications, p. 253.

important, and for this reason, I have recommended natural woodblock sounds, rather than electronic beeping.

Manaka demonstrated that different channels respond to different frequencies, and by switching off the metronome and applying Ontake unaccompanied, we can reduce the dosage considerably, removing two separate streams of stimulation at the proprioceptive and auditory levels.

We can summarise this discussion by saying that the effect of Ontake is comprised of three unequal components. In my opinion, they can be ordered in importance: heat, frequency, then technique. This can be represented below in the following impressionistic proportions:

Components of Ontake Effects

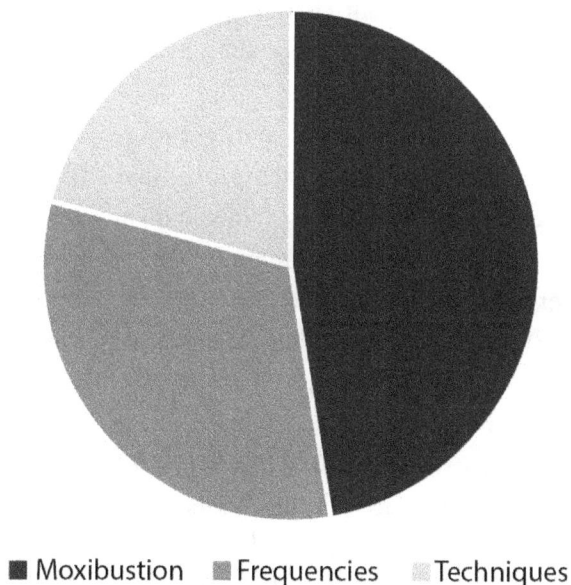

■ Moxibustion ■ Frequencies ▦ Techniques

Planning a Treatment and Sticking to It

As practitioners of acupuncture, moxibustion, and other meridian therapies, we have an extensive repertoire of techniques and methods to choose from when treating both the root and the branch. We have seen Manaka's analogy that root treatment and branch treatment are like the wheels on the front axle of a car. When treating elderly or sensitive patients, therefore, it makes sense to plan your treatments very carefully.

If you are going to do a strong root treatment, then plan to do less branch treatment. If you plan to do a major branch treatment, make sure it fits in with your assessment of the patient's sensitivity. For example, *shiraku* (bloodletting) should only be used with extreme care on sensitive patients.

Stephen Birch has emphasised in lectures that what you plan to do should be decided upon and mapped out in your mind before you insert your first needle. It's easy to make mistakes if you simply try out one technique after another. Successful treatment is the harmonious planning and combination of different elements and methods.

Mr Takai also explained in lectures that when patients present with many diverse symptoms, we should focus only on root treatment. This is a critical point to consider. Some patients arrive with a long shopping list of symptoms, thinking that there is an acupuncture point that should be needled for each one. This is Western thinking: take one drug for this symptom, take a second drug for the next one, and take a third drug for the side effects of taking the first two. In TEAM thinking, where there are many symptoms, it is much better to focus on root treatment.

As patients get stronger, you can change the emphasis of treatment over time. Start with root treatment and gradually introduce branch treatment for one particular symptom.

Another consideration is that some patients get more demanding at the end of a session and request that you treat various symptoms that still remain.

"Can you do anything for my shoulder? Did you do anything for my knee today?"

In my experience, it is often at this moment, when trying to please them, that my treatments slip out of the Goldilocks Zone into overtreatment. Armed with bamboo, pain relief can be so easy to achieve, so I start to chase symptoms. At this late stage in the session, strange reactions then occur, so I have to fix them, just like prescribing a drug to counteract the side effects of the first two.

To stay in the Zone, it is essential to be firm and maintain boundaries with demanding patients. Many patients, despite years of other therapies that have not worked, expect that acupuncture should work in forty-five minutes. It is good to explain to them that it reaches its peak effect after two or three days, so they need to wait and see. Most patients will settle down if you explain the concept of overtreatment.

Putting It All Together

In my practice, Ontake is used much less often as the sole modality and much more often as an add-on technique. Thus, when planning a treatment, the dosage of Ontake needs to be considered within the context of all the other things I plan to do. One of my first teachers of acupuncture, German trainer Barbara Kirschbaum, used a delightful analogy for treatment, comparing it to making soup. When you make soup, you taste it from time to time, adding a little salt here, a bit of spice there.

Treatment is a combination of similar flavours, but you need to be aware of the dosimeter and how the patient is reacting to each new taste. In practical terms, keep taking the pulse and palpating the skin. The three principal warning signs that you are leaving the Goldilocks Zone are when the pulse loses definition, becomes more superficial or if the skin gets moist. Close down the treatment with some Ontake at DU 14 or stop treatment altogether.

While we are on the subject of dosage, we can review how to moderate the dosage across a wide variety of techniques.

Table 12. Moderating Dosage

Method or Technique	Description	Moderation
Point selection		• Select fewer points. • Treat unilaterally.
Polarity methods	Positive and negative polarities are applied to the skin, using north and south magnets, ion-pumping cords, ion-beam devices, electrostatic adsorbers, copper and zinc buttons, copper and zinc needles, or gold and silver needles.	• Use fewer pairs • Maintain polarity for a shorter time.
Retained needle	Needles are inserted and left in place.	• Use finer needles. • Reduce insertion depth. • Reduce manipulation and needle sensation. • Retain for less time.
Warm needle	Moxa is burnt on the needle handle.	• Use finer moxa that burns at a lower temperature. • Use smaller balls of moxa. • Use longer needles or insert less deeply so that moxa is further from the skin. • Use fewer balls.

Touch needling (*sesshokushin*)	A specialised Toyohari acupuncture method, here a needle is held on the skin without insertion. The practitioner uses intention and changing the grip of the fingers of the left hand on the needle to move qi.	• Use fewer points. • Use less intention and less closure of the left hand. • Use a finer silver needle. • Use a *teishin* instead of a needle.
Direct Moxibustion	Large or small cones of moxa are burnt directly on the skin: • *Tonnetsukyu*: The cones are burnt until the patient feels heat. • *Chinetsukyu*: The cones are burnt until the patient feels warmth or removed before.	• Select fewer points. • Do not allow the patient to feel heat. • Do not allow the patient to feel warmth.
Cupping	Cups are placed on the skin, and some of the air is removed. The reduced pressure sucks up the underlying tissue engorging the area.	• Use fewer cups. • Retain for a shorter time. • Use less suction.
Shiraku (bloodletting)	Points are pricked and squeezed for the therapeutic release of blood. Wet Cupping: Areas are needled several times then cupped to cause minor bleeding under the cup.	• Use with great caution on sensitive patients. Reduce the number of points to 1 and squeeze just 1 or 2 drops. • Wet cupping should be avoided on sensitive patients.
Ontake	Heated bamboo is applied at specific frequencies of beats per minute.	• Reduce treatment time. • Use lighter methods. • Turn off the metronome.

Conclusion

It is the natural urge of every healer to want to help as much as possible. It is also the natural urge of most patients to try and get as much bang for their buck as they can. These two drives can conspire against successful treatment. Enough is better than too much.

Recalling 90 percent of adverse reactions in Mr Takai's practice were due to overtreatment, it seems that incorporating the concept of the Goldilocks Zone is the single most important thing you can do to reduce the risk of things going wrong in your practice. Even so, once you have the concept in your head, it takes a long time to integrate it. As can be seen from the table above, adjusting dosage is a very delicate, multifaceted task, and you have to keep engaged throughout the session— like a master chef tasting her soup throughout the preparation.

Mr Murakami, a senior instructor in the Toyohari Association, explained that we want to bring our patients from Point A, the starting point, to Point Z, the finish line during a course of treatment. It is in our eager human nature to want to get patients there as fast as possible. Nevertheless, we should be quite content if we go only from A to F in one session. We can always continue from F in the next session.

On top of twenty-first century cultural expectations that results should be instant, it seems that there is also a constant struggle between our temptation to give more and our duty to give less. When I am tempted to do too much, it is with Mr Murakami's simple wisdom that I can comfort myself and strengthen my resolve to limit my treatments.

Summary

This chapter introduced several key concepts for effective practice:
- Each patient has a Goldilocks Zone of treatment that is neither too much nor too little—but just right.
- Effective treatment is about knowing how much treatment is enough for a particular patient on a given day.

This requires identifying sensitive and robust patients with your inner jitsometer and moderating treatment accordingly.

We have now covered how to treat at the root and branch levels with Ontake and how to moderate the dosage of treatment throughout the session. In the next section, we go beyond what was previously possible with bamboo and look at its most interesting application: integrating meridian frequency moxibustion with holographic theory for the rapid relief of pain.

PART 3

GOING HOLOGRAPHIC

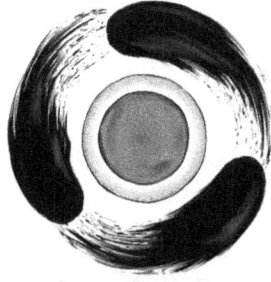

CHAPTER 11

ONTAKE 1, 2, 3—PAIN RELIEF

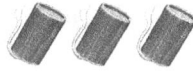

Integrating various holographic models with the tension assessment and traditional channel pairings to provide rapid pain relief with Ontake.

Describing the work of Dr Tan and how his ideas can be adapted to treat pain with Ontake.

Holographic Systems

The word Taiji has been applied to medicine by many classical physicians, and several writers describe the body as being comprised of numerous "Taiji holograms... Taiji means that all properties—or in modern parlance, all information—of the whole body is also contained in its individual parts and vice versa. Consequently, each part of the body can influence every other part through its anatomical and functional relationships with the whole organism.

—McCann and Ross[111]

111 McCann, H., & Ross, H. (2015). *Practical Atlas of Tung's Acupuncture*. Germany: Verlag Muller & Steinicke, p. 15.

A single human zygote contains all the genetic information necessary to create a whole person. If everything that we are comes from just one cell, then structural elements in adults can be traced back topographically to structures in embryonic cells. This was the lynchpin idea of Manaka's octahedral model, which describes how the eight extraordinary vessels are formed in the first three divisions of the human zygote. The zygote divides into two, four, then eight cells, and these eight cells contain the three axes and the eight surfaces of the octahedron. These aspects are retained in our adult form.[112]

It is from these ideas that we can begin to understand holographic theory: the idea that every small part of the body contains the information of the whole. A hologram is defined as "a three-dimensional image of a given object which contains the information of the object in itself and in every part of itself".[113]

One of the fundamental ideas of Chinese medicine is that humans occupy the physical space between heaven and earth. Chinese medicine assumes a unity between each organism and its environment, between inner and outer: "This philosophy of unity is described as Heaven, Earth and Humanity in Harmony."[114] The concept of holographic and microacupuncture systems takes this idea further, assuming that each part of the body is a microcosm of the whole.

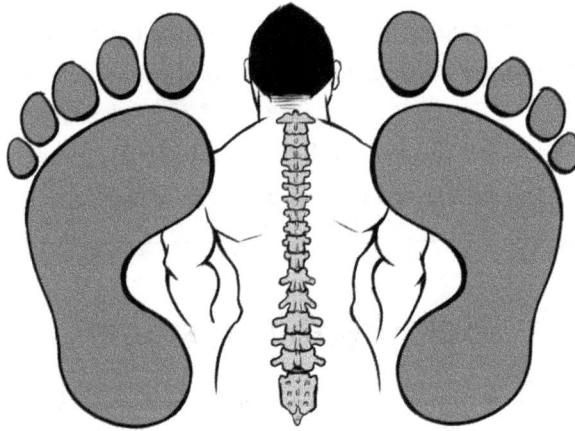

Possibly the most famous holographic system of all is
reflexology: your feet reflect your body.

112   Manaka, Y., Itaya, K., & Birch, S. (1995). *Chasing the Dragon's Tail: The Theory and Practice of Acupuncture in the Work of Yoshio Manaka*. Brookline: Paradigm Publications.

113   Dale, R. (1999). The Systems, Holograms and Theory of Micro-Acupuncture. *American Journal of Acupuncture, 27*(3-4), 207–42.

114   McCann, H., & Ross, H., (2015). *Practical Atlas of Tung's Acupuncture*. Germany: Verlag Muller & Steinicke, p. 17.

Possibly the most famous of all microcosms or holographic systems is foot reflexology. In Asia, reflexology salons are found in every mall and high street. They're staffed by practitioners who tell you, with varying degrees of accuracy, where you are sick by pressing painful points on your feet. The feet are a hologram of the body: the upper part of the body reflects in the toes, the lower part in the heels, and the two medial surfaces of the feet when joined together, reflect the midline and spine.

Less well known to the general public are the holographic systems taught in every acupuncture school. The most obvious microcosm of the body that we consider daily is the tongue. The tip corresponds to the upper burner (the upper part of the body); the middle to the organs of digestion in the middle burner; and the root to the organs of elimination in the lower burner. Once again, the trinity of Heaven, Humanity, and Earth is reflected in the structure of the three burners.

Another hologram of the body, only evident through palpation, is the pulse. Once again, the pulse can be taken in three positions (upper, middle and lower), corresponding to the upper, middle, and lower parts of the body.

Two other familiar holographic systems are the front-*mu* point and back-*shu* point groupings. Unlike the ear, which is a miniaturised acupuncture system that reflects the macro-anatomy, the back-*shu* points are on a one to one scale. The upper points reflect and treat the upper part of the body, the middle points reflect and treat the middle part of the body, and the lower points reflect and treat the lower part of the body. Anatomically, these represent the organs and are used both diagnostically and therapeutically.[115] The back-*shu* points can be thought of as a conceptual bridge between traditional acupuncture ideas and more modern holographic thinking.[116]

In Japanese acupuncture, *fukushin* (diagnosing by abdominal palpation) has become a fine art that uses information in the abdominal hologram of the body. Manaka took traditional mappings further and charted reaction lines for the Eight Extras onto the *hara* (abdomen). By doing so, he mapped his own octahedral model.

Some holograms, such as the tongue, are used for diagnosis only, but others can be used therapeutically. The first microacupuncture system to be fully developed was that of the ear, discovered by Paul Nogier in the 1950s. The ear contains a miniaturised system of acupuncture points that have systemic effects on the body.

Since Nogier, many other new holographic systems have been discovered and developed. Microacupuncture systems have been researched on the foot, face, nose, hand, finger, scalp, wrist, ankle, teeth, lips and philtrum. Each of these demonstrates

---

115   Dale, R. (1999). The Systems, Holograms and Theory of Micro-Acupuncture. *American Journal of Acupuncture, 27*(3-4), 207–42.

116   Hecker, H., Steveling, A., & Peuker, E. (2005). *Microsystems Acupuncture: The Complete Guide: Ear-Scalp-Mouth-Hand.* Stuttgart: Thieme, p. XIV.

the same relationship between the overall macro-anatomy and the topology of the micro-acupoints.

Balance Method and Dr Tan

The range and scope of Ontake treatment can be broadened considerably by the integration of the holographic models used by the late Dr Richard Teh Fu Tan. These models provide an additional framework for applying bamboo for the rapid relief of pain.

Before Dr Tan passed away in 2015, he was a highly effective Chinese practitioner and teacher who popularised a simple approach to balancing yin and yang. Not only did he use the dynamic relationships between different pairings of meridians to balance the body, he also used holographic and isophasal relationships (see below) between different areas of the body to select the best areas to needle.

The five systems of pairing channels and holographic mappings may sound familiar to practitioners of Master Tung's acupuncture, because Dr Tan studied Master Tung's work extensively. However, Dr Tan's approach was principally influenced by the balancing methods derived from the Ba Gua described by Dr Chao Chen,[117] and it is likely that Dr Tan's approach was a synthesis of these ideas and others—an attempt to simplify them and make them more accessible to a Western acupuncture audience.[118]

The hologram concepts in this chapter are taken straight from Dr Tan's book *Acupuncture 1, 2, 3*, but it is worth acknowledging that no teacher of Dr Tan's Balance Method or Master Tung's acupuncture has ever used or endorsed Ontake warm bamboo. What follows is my own integration of these ideas into an effective system of pain relief with bamboo. It follows that any mistakes, misrepresentations, or deviations from orthodoxy concerning these two remarkable styles of acupuncture are my own: by design, because that is how I find Ontake works best, or as a product of my own misunderstanding.

Acupuncture One, Two, Three

First described in his book *Acupuncture 1, 2, 3,* Dr Tan called his treatment the Balance Method.[119] The idea is very simple. If you can identify which channel is out of balance, you can rectify it by treating its natural pair. For example, if the bladder

117   Chen, C. (1975). *Essence of Acupuncture Therapy as Based on Yi King and Computers.* Taiwan: International Acupuncture Congress.

118   Tan, R. T. (2007). *Acupuncture 1, 2, 3.* San Diego, CA: R. Tan.

119   Ibid.

channel is sick, then the balancing channel could be the kidney. Dr Tan described and used five pairings, which he named Systems 1–5.

His book describes a three-step protocol. First, we have to identify the "sick" meridian. In the context of Ontake, we are using Balance Method concepts simply for pain relief, so this first step is quite simple: the sick channel is generally where it hurts. Next, we have to figure out which paired meridian balances the sick channel best. Finally, we use one of Dr Tan's holographic mappings to decide the area to needle.

From the description above, Dr Tan's method may not yet seem very remarkable. Most acupuncturists know that channels are paired in various ways and that these pairings can be exploited for treatment. What is special about using channel pairings? Well, what makes his system so effective is that he overlays these basic pairings with holographic thinking. These holographic mappings dictate where on the paired channel to needle, and by putting the two systems together, he created something new and significantly more effective.

Dr Tan's protocol works extremely well for both channel and organ problems, but it can involve deep needling, sometimes right down to the bone, often with many needles. If the pain changes location, more needling may be necessary on a new paired channel.

With some simple adaptations and stripping down the theory to use only three systems of meridian pairings, Ontake can be used for pain relief in exactly the same way. In my own practice, it achieves equivalent results very rapidly, and yet it feels very comfortable to receive. Because bamboo is so mobile, the user can adapt to changes in pain location very easily.

Dr Tan's Holographic Models

Terminology

Dr Tan developed terminology that should be used in a very specific way.
- **Mirroring** describes the relationship between the left arm and the right arm, the left leg and the right leg, and the upper limb and the lower limb.
- **Imaging** describes the relationship between the torso and the upper and lower limb, and the relationship between the head and the upper and lower limb.

These are two distinctly different kinds of holograms, and the terms should not be confused or used interchangeably.

The Normal Mirror

Dr Manaka coined the term "isophasal". He used it to describe parts of the body that have the same signature or resonance. For example, the earth points on the liver channel are isophasal with other earth points. The lumbar area on the ear microsystem is isophasal with the lumbar area in Korean hand acupuncture and, of course, with the lumbar area itself. A ball and socket joint is isophasal with other ball and socket joints.

While the left arm clearly mirrors the right, and the right leg mirrors the left, what is less obvious is the relationship between the upper limb and the lower limb.

The upper limb and lower limb are isophasal: they have similar, resonating structures. For example, the ball and socket joint of the shoulder is structurally identical to the ball and socket joint of the hip, the humerus is a single long bone like the femur, and both the elbow and knee have hinge joints. Likewise, the forearm and lower leg contain two long bones that connect to smaller carpal and tarsal bones in the wrist and ankle, which then open up to metacarpal and metatarsal bones, then the fingers and toes.

Without ever using Manaka's specific term, Tan's concept of mirroring exploits this isophasality so that you can use the shoulder to treat the hip, the elbow to treat the knee, the wrist to treat the ankle or vice versa. By the same token, you can use the right arm to treat the left, the right leg to treat the left, or vice versa.

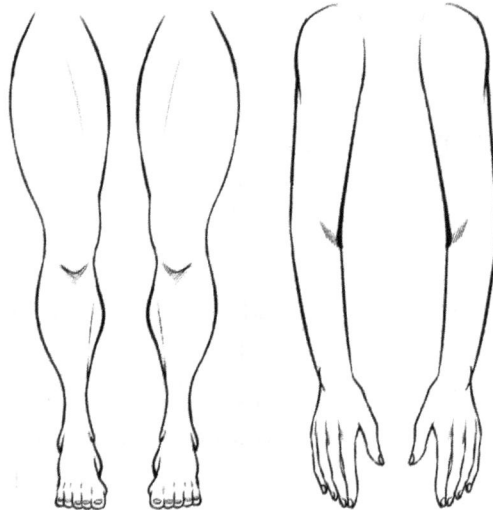

The left and right limbs are mirrors of each other.

Table 13. Left and Right Mirroring on the Arm

Left Arm Treats Right	Right Arm Treats Left
Shoulder	Shoulder
Upper arm	Upper arm
Elbow	Elbow
Forearm	Forearm
Wrist	Wrist
Hand	Hand
Fingers	Fingers

Table 14. Left and Right Mirroring on the Leg

Left Leg Treats Right	Right Leg Treats Left
Hip	Hip
Thigh	Thigh
Knee	Knee
Lower leg	Lower leg
Ankle	Ankle
Foot	Foot
Toes	Toes

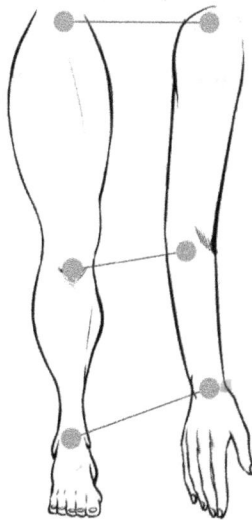

The upper and lower limbs are mirrors of each other.

Table 15. Upper Limb and Lower Limb Mirroring

Upper Limb	Lower Limb
Shoulder	Hip
Upper arm	Thigh
Elbow	Knee
Forearm	Lower leg
Wrist	Ankle
Hand	Foot
Fingers	Toes

The Reverse Mirror

The normal mirror concepts above are easy to follow and have been discussed in Chinese acupuncture books since the 1960s.[120] What is less easy to grasp is Dr Tan's concept of the reverse mirror. It's a system of reverse correspondences.

To visualise how you can use the reverse mirror to treat the left arm with the right, imagine putting your hand on top of a friend's shoulder. With your hand resting over the shoulder, your fingers, thumb and palm wrap around it. Your wrist joint is now lying on top of the shoulder joint. Your forearm is lying adjacent to the upper arm. The midpoint of both arms is the elbow. Your upper arm now pairs with your model's forearm. Your shoulder pairs up with the wrist, and your shoulder blade matches your friend's hand. With this reverse mapping, if you want to treat pain in the shoulder joint, you can look for reactions at the wrist joint.

---

120   Bensky D., O'Connor, J, (1996). *Acupuncture–A Comprehensive Text,* Shanghai, College of Traditional Medicine Hardcover.

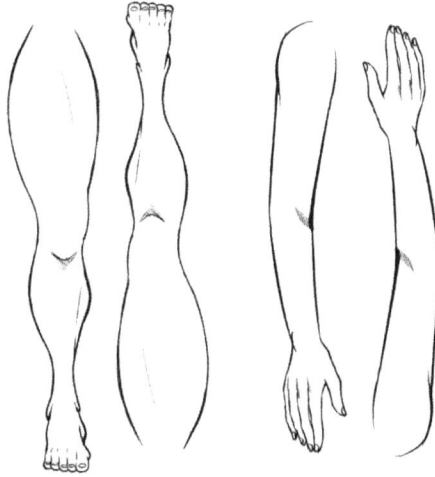

Left and right reverse mirrors.

Table 16. Reverse Mirror on the Upper Limb

Left Arm Treats Right	Right Arm Treats Left
Shoulder	Hand and fingers
Shoulder joint	Wrist joint
Upper arm	Forearm
Elbow	Elbow
Forearm	Upper arm
Wrist joint	Shoulder joint
Hand and fingers	Shoulder

Table 17. Reverse Mirror on the Lower Limb

Left Leg Treats Right	Right Leg Treats Left
Hip	Foot and toes
Hip joint	Ankle joint
Thigh	Lower leg
Knee	Knee
Lower leg	Thigh
Ankle	Hip joint
Feet and toes	Hip

You can also use the reverse mirror to map the arm on the leg and vice versa. Unless you actually have one, imagine holding an Action Man or a Barbie doll and—purely in the interest of science—pull off one leg! Maybe you have an acupuncturist's doll, with the channel pathways etched on it. Pull off an arm! Now place the foot over the shoulder blade. The ankle joint corresponds to the shoulder joint. The lower leg matches the upper arm and the knee the elbow. The thigh now matches the forearm, the hip joint matches the wrist, and finally the hip matches the hand and fingers.

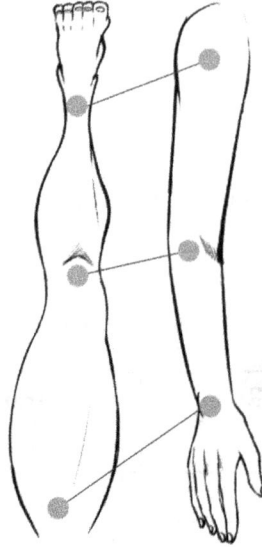

Upper and lower limb reverse mirror

Table 18. Reverse Mirror on the Upper and Lower Limb

Upper limb	Lower limb
Shoulder	Toes, foot
Shoulder joint	Ankle joint
Upper arm	Lower leg
Elbow	Knee
Forearm	Thigh
Wrist	Hip joint
Hand	Hip
Fingers	Top of hip

What is interesting to note is that whether you use the normal or reverse mirror, the elbow always corresponds to the knee.

The Normal Image

Holographic theory states that each part of the whole reflects and encodes the information of the whole. We have seen that the arm is a hologram of the leg and vice versa. The arm and leg are also hologrammatic representations of the torso and head.

In the two illustrations below, the trunk, from the top of head to the genitalia, can be mapped out from the top of the shoulder to the fingers and from the top of the hips to the toes.

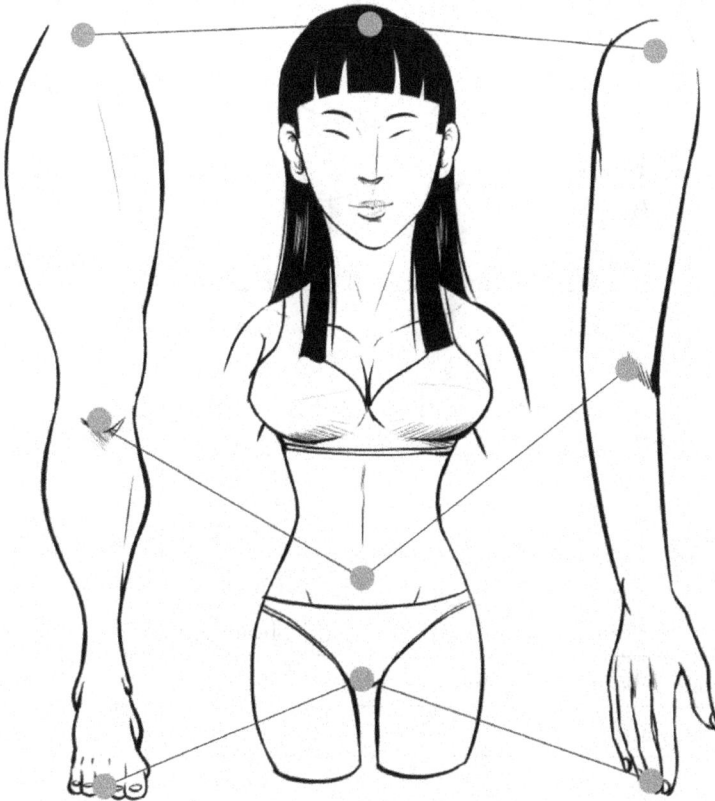

The normal image of the torso (front).

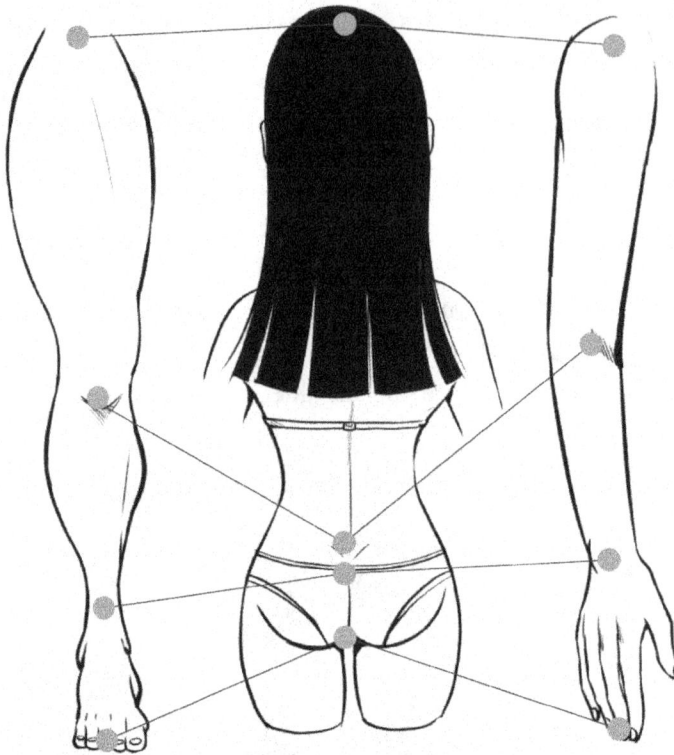

The normal image of the torso (back).

Table 19. Torso (Normal Image)

Image	Upper Limb	Lower Limb
Area Affected	Ontake Area	Ontake Area
Top of the head	Top of the shoulder	Top of the hip
Neck, jaw, base of skull	Shoulder joint	Hip joint
Upper abdomen, ribcage, chest, mid-upper back	Upper arm	Upper leg
Umbilicus, L-2, waist	Elbow	Knee
Lower abdomen, lower back	Forearm	Lower leg
L-5/S-1, genitals, bladder, sacrum	Wrist joint	Ankle joint
Genitals, lower sacrum, coccyx	Hand	Foot
Testicles, anus	Fingers	Toes

Columns 2 and 3 are the areas where you apply stimulation (in our case, with Ontake), and column 1 is where the effect is felt. When you want to treat the top of the head, you apply Ontake to the top of the shoulder or the top of the hip. Once again, it is interesting to note the importance of the elbow and knee area, both reflecting the umbilicus and L-2, where the body hinges.

The Reverse Image

Just like the reverse mirror for the limbs, described previously, Dr Tan used a reverse image for the torso. To visualise this, hold your forearm up and let your hand flop forwards. Imagine a glove puppet, with your hand as the head and your wrist as the neck. Animate the puppet and move your hand around.*[121] If you understand this image, make your hand nod! If you still don't understand this image, make it shake its head!

If you are one of those flexible practitioners, you can also lift up your leg and pretend that your foot is your head and your ankle your neck. Can you see how the Achilles tendon is isophasal with the trapezius, below the occiput? Nod your foot, to show you understand! Below are the correspondences for the reverse image.

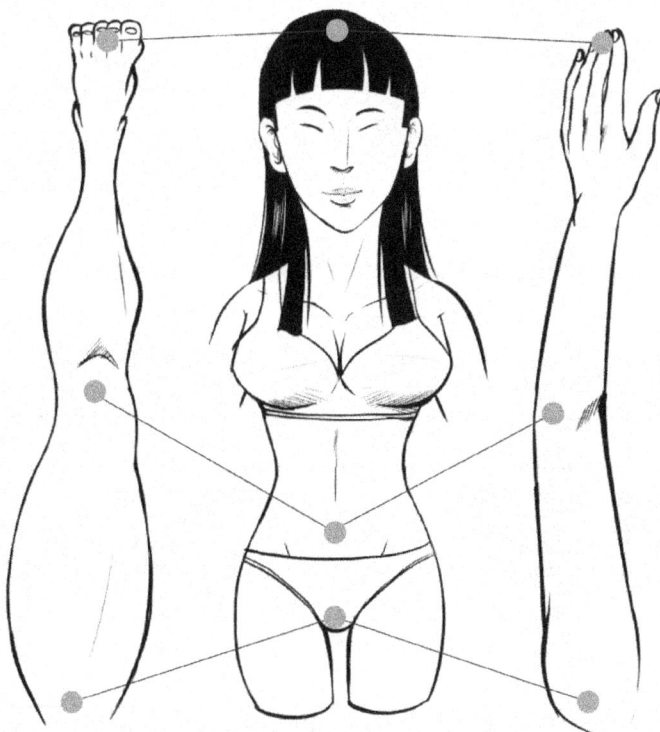

The reverse image of the torso (front).

---

*121 This delightful image of a glove puppet comes from my teacher of the Balance Method in the UK, Ekaterina (Katia) Fedotova.

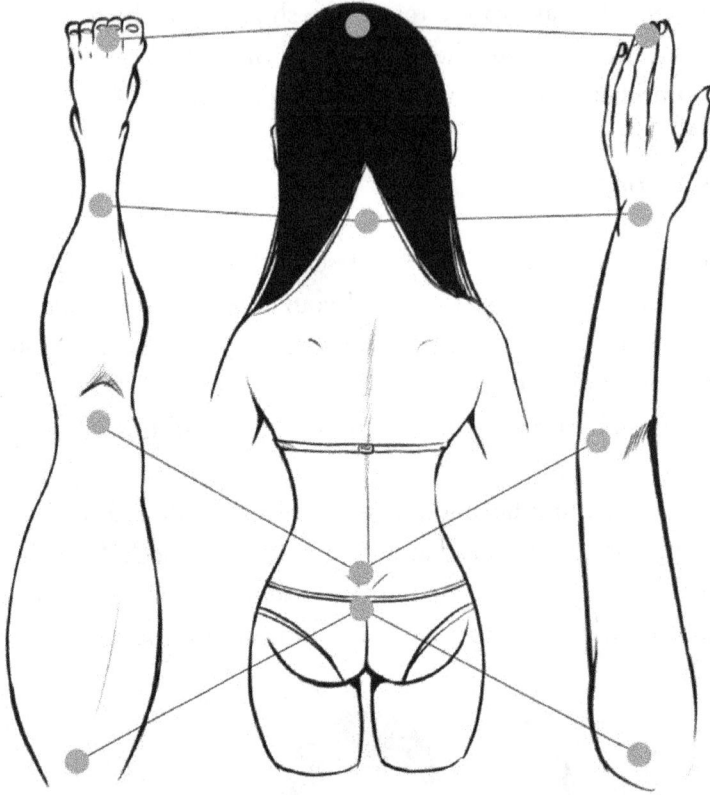

The reverse image of the torso (back).

Table 20. Torso Reverse Image

Image	Upper Limb	Lower Limb
Area Affected	Ontake Area	Ontake Area
Testicles, anus	Top of the shoulder	Top of the hip
L-5/S-1 Sacrum, coccyx, genitals	Shoulder joint	Hip joint
Lower abdomen, lower back	Upper arm	Upper leg
Umbilicus, L-2, waist	Elbow	Knee
Upper abdomen, ribcage, chest and mid-upper back	Forearm	Lower leg
Neck and neck joints	Wrist	Ankle
Head and base of skull	Hand	Foot
Top of the head	Finger	Toe

Head Mappings

The head can also be mapped out on the upper and lower limb. Once again, this can be done with a normal image and a reversed image. Below you can see the isophasal relationship between the hinge joints of the elbow, knee, and jaw.

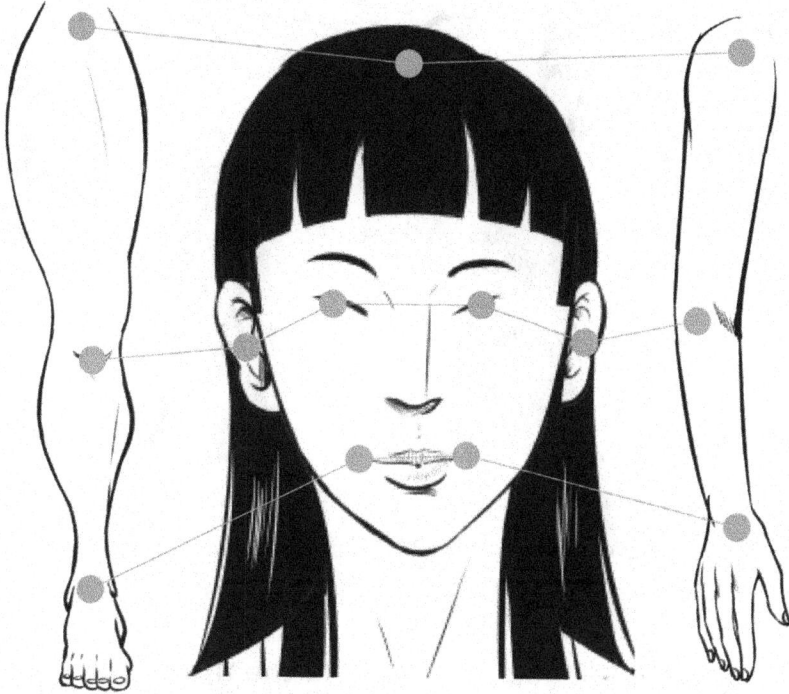

Normal image of head to upper and lower limb.

Table 21. Normal Image of the Head to the Upper and Lower Limb

Image	Upper Limb	Lower Limb
Area Affected	Ontake Area	Ontake Area
Top of the head	Shoulder joint	Hip joint
Forehead level	Upper arm	Upper leg
Eye, ear, occiput	Elbow	Knee
Nose level	Forearm	Lower leg
Mouth level	Wrist, hand	Ankle, foot
Chin level	Fingers	Toes

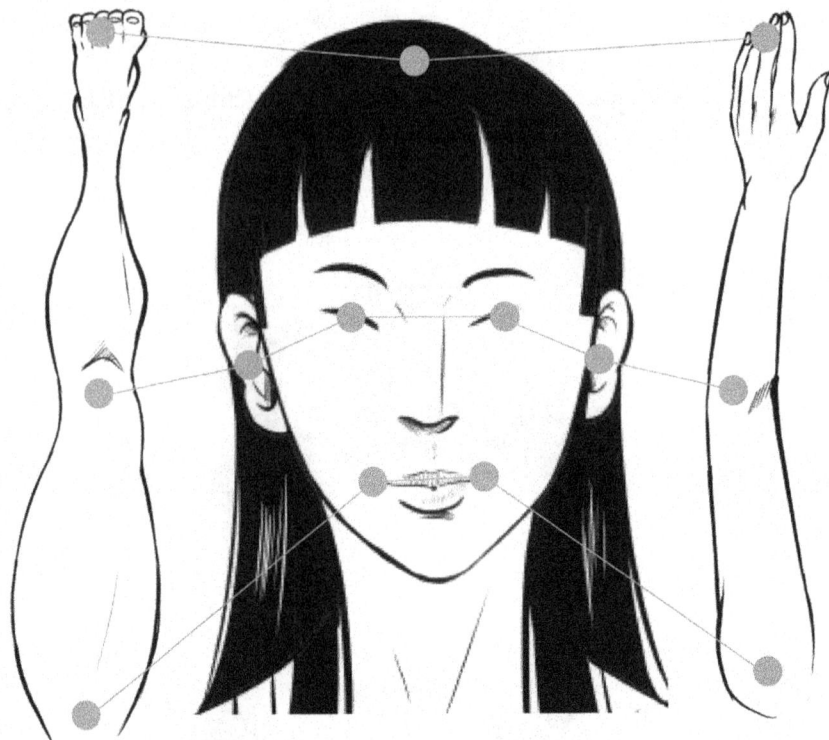

Reverse image of head to upper and lower limb.

Table 22. Reverse Image of the Head to the Upper and Lower Limb

Image	Upper Limb	Lower Limb
Area Affected	Ontake Area	Ontake Area
Top of the head	Fingers	Toes
Between the forehead, the top of the head	Wrist, hand	Ankle, foot
Forehead level	Forearm	Lower leg
Eye, ear, occiput	Elbow	Knee
Nose level	Upper arm	Upper leg
Mouth level	Shoulder	Hip
Chin level	Shoulder joint	Hip joint

Choosing Orientation

Which orientation works best, and why would you select one over the other? My impression is that Dr Tan was very pragmatic: "Points should be chosen according to effectiveness, efficiency and convenience".[122]

He liked to treat his patients as they sat upright rather than having them lie down. He also preferred they remain dressed rather than undress. This means that the points below the elbows and knees get priority. Moreover, these points are the most dynamic, being the furthest out from the centre. This would mean that when treating the head, you would tend to choose the reverse image, and when treating the lower back and sacrum, you would use the normal image. However, Dr Tan also stated that "typically, straightforward imaging and mirror relations are used more frequently than reverse imaging and mirror concepts".[123]

In the case of Ontake, the application is different. Firstly, although it is preferable to apply Ontake directly on the skin, it can be used through clothing, especially if your patient's shirt or blouse is thin, so practical concerns about accessibility are not as relevant. Secondly, unlike with needling, it is easy to change strategies and switch orientations when using Ontake, so if a normal orientation is not working well, you might investigate and treat the opposite end of the limb.

Some areas are isophasal to others. For example, in the glove puppet reverse image orientation of the arm, you can see that the tendons of the wrist bear a similarity to the thick muscles of the neck, so there is an isophasal resonance between the wrist and neck that might make this orientation better. The same is true for the Achilles tendon, which is isophasal to the back of the neck and top of trapezius. Sometimes it makes sense to treat the neck from the wrist because of this isophasal resonance. For me, orientation selection is guided mostly by palpation and looking for reactions. These reactions become more predictable the more I use the system. Palpation and observation should tell you where to treat more reliably than theory.

Pairings

All acupuncture styles use channel pairings. In MSA and Toyohari, three pairing systems are used: internal/external, six-channel pairs, and *shigo* (polar channel pairs). Dr Tan's Balance Method uses five systems of channel pairings, and when diagnosing, these five balancing channel options are organised into a grid Dr Tan called the Systems Matrix. Practitioners of the Balance Method who read this chapter are more

122 Tan, R. T. (2007). *Acupuncture 1, 2, 3*. San Diego, CA: R. Tan, p. 153.
123 Ibid.

than welcome to use all five systems with Ontake, but for clarity and simplicity, I have kept this discussion to the three I have found most useful. Ontake has proven very effective with just these three. For some readers, these pairings are second nature, but for others, reiterating these concepts from the perspective of classical acupuncture may be useful.

Table 23. Pairing Systems with Ontake

System	Name	Explanation
1	Internal / External	Five phase interior/exterior relationships, such as the lung and the large intestine.
2	Six-Channel Pairs	Refers to hand and foot pairings according to six channels, also known as the Six Divisions (e.g., hand and foot *taiyin*, lung and spleen).
3	*Shigo* (Polar Channel Pairs)	Polar channel pairs according to Chinese clock/midday-midnight (e.g., kidney/large intestine, heart/gall bladder, lung/bladder). Dr Tan called this relationship Clock Opposites.

Internal and External Pairings

Every yin meridian has its yang opposite. The yin meridians are grouped along the anterior medial aspects of the limbs, and the yang channels are on the posterior lateral aspects. Yin channels tend to become *kyo*, and yang channels tend to become *jitsu*. Thus, this pairing is the most fundamental way of balancing yin and yang.

The three arm yin channels are paired to the three arm yang channels. The three leg yin channels are paired to the three leg yang channels.

Table 24. Internal/External Channel Pairings

Element	Upper/Lower	Yin	Yang
Metal	Arm	Lung	Large intestine
Fire	Arm	Pericardium	Triple burner
Fire	Arm	Heart	Small intestine
Earth	Leg	Spleen	Stomach
Wood	Leg	Liver	Gall bladder
Water	Leg	Kidney	Bladder

These pairings derive from Five Phase (Five Element) theory. Each phase has one pair (except fire, which has two).

Six Channels (Six Divisions)

In the internal/external pairings above, each pair is either on the arm or on the leg; for example, the lung and large intestine both traverse the arm. Each of the six hand channels can also be paired with one of the six leg channels, according to the amount of yin or yang circulating in that part of the body. Dr Tan simply says that "Yang areas generally refer to body parts that are exposed more to the sun than Yin areas. ... Yin areas generally refer to body parts that are exposed less to the sun than Yang areas.[124]

If you stand with your arms by your sides, these paired channels on your arms and legs share anatomical similarities, relating to the amount of yin or yang circulating there. For example, the most anterior of the yang channels on the arm and leg are the large intestine and stomach channels; the ones on the median lateral line on the arm and leg are the triple burner and gall bladder channels; and the ones on the posterior yang aspect are the small intestine and bladder channels.

To visualise this, hold out your right hand, palm facing down. Now place your left hand on your right wrist so that your left index finger is resting on the ulnar at the small intestine channel (SI 6). If you now rotate your wrist so that your right palm faces up, you'll see that your left index finger traverses first the three yang channels (small intestine, triple burner, and large intestine) and then the three yin channels lung, pericardium to rest on heart (hand *shaoyin*).

You can repeat the movement on the leg by resting the index finger of your left hand under your left thigh, just posterior to BL 40. If you trace a transverse circle clockwise around your thigh, your finger will traverse the bladder, gall bladder, stomach, spleen, and liver to rest on the kidney (foot *shaoyin*). This circle connects with each channel in the same order as on the arm.

This six-channel theory appeared in the *Shang Han Lun (Discussion of Cold-Induced Disorders)* by Zhang Zhong Jing to describe the progression of fevers from the outside to the inside. In this context, we are discussing each channel in terms of its position on the body, not by its related organ name. For example, the lung is described as hand *taiyin*, and the bladder is foot *taiyang*. Some commentators even go so far as to describe these pairings as one channel, so that large intestine and stomach are thought of as one entity: the *yangming* channel.

---

124   Tan, R. T. (2007). *Acupuncture 1, 2, 3*. San Diego, CA: R. Tan, p. 1.

Table 25 Six channel pairings

Name	Aspect	Meaning	Hand	Foot
Taiyang	Outer	Greater Yang	Small Intestine	Bladder
Shaoyang	Middle	Lesser Yang	Triple Burner	Gall Bladder
Yangming	Inner	Bright Yang	Large Intestine	Stomach
Taiyin	Outer	Greater Yin	Lung	Spleen
Jueyin	Middle	Terminal Yin	Pericardium	Liver
Shaoyin	Inner	Lesser Yin	Heart	Kidney

In terms of Ontake treatment for pain, these positional relationships are significant.

Shigo (Polar Channel Pairs)

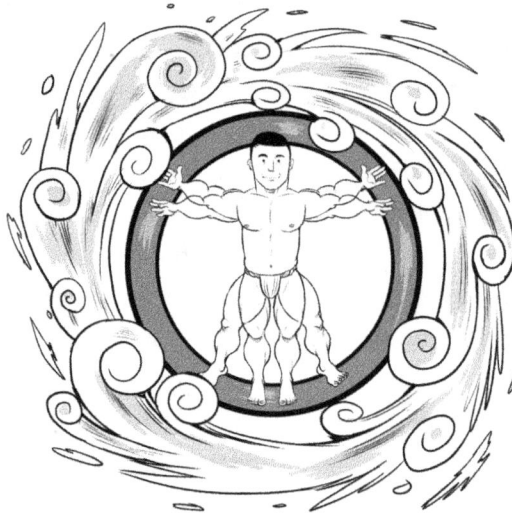

The *Nai Zhi Fa* describes the twenty-four-hour cycle of
energy as a slow-moving wave.

Nai Zhi Fa, or the Twenty-Four-Hour Cycle

The last pairing arises from a theoretical concept in TEAM that lends itself to many different clinical applications. The Chinese Clock, or *Nai Zhi Fa*, describes a slow movement of energy throughout the channels, surging like a wave in slow-motion. This wave moves through the channel system over a twenty-four-hour period, a rolling surge of energy every two hours in one of the twelve channels. This rolling surge connects paired channels from the two systems above to make its way through the channel system (see pie chart). Every two hours, one channel peaks as the swelling wave enters and makes its way through it.

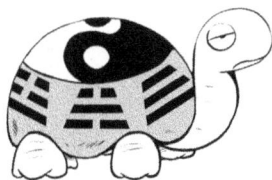

This surge is so slow that we can imagine it more as a well-fed "qi turtle" crawling slowly up and down the channels. The peak surge in the channels is wherever the little turtle has reached. It sets off from LU 1 on a twenty-four-hour journey, taking over two hours to glide down your arm to your thumb. Next, it has another two hours to reach LI 20 at the side of your nose. To visualise this, we can trace its trajectory on our own bodies with a finger, or even better, with an Ontake.

Roll the Ontake or trace your index finger along the hand-*taiyin*-lung channel from LU 1 to LU 11. Then cross over to the internal-external pair, hand-*yangming*-large intestine. From LI 1, trace your finger along the hand-*yangming*-large intestine to LI 20, then cross to stomach-foot-*yangming* at ST 1. From ST 1, trace the stomach channel down the torso, thigh, and leg to ST 45, then cross over to the foot-*taiyin* spleen channel at SP 1. From SP 1 trace the spleen channel back up the leg until you reach SP 21.

Manaka described this group of four channels as a four-channel set and enthusiastically set about testing their relationships with north and south magnets. He was able to demonstrate that channels in a four-channel set can have significant influences on each other.[125] The next four-channel set is heart–small intestine–bladder-kidney, once again moving from chest to hand to head to foot to chest. The final set is pericardium–triple burner–gall bladder–liver.

The Chinese Clock

The Chinese clock is a twenty-four-hour clock divided into twelve two-hour segments and can be represented graphically in various ways. Below we can see that each time segment has a channel associated with it, and that the same time twelve hours later has a different channel, thus creating a pair.

---

125   Manaka, Y., Itaya, K., & Birch, S. (1995). *Chasing the Dragon's Tail: The Theory and Practice of Acupuncture in the Work of Yoshio Manaka*. Brookline: Paradigm Publications, pp. 60–65.

Table 26. Clock Pairings

Time	Channel	Polar Channel
3-5	Lung	Bladder
5-7	Large Intestine	Kidney
7-9	Stomach	Pericardium
9-11	Spleen	Triple Heater
11-1	Heart	Gall bladder
1-3	Small Intestine	Liver

Looking at the pairings chart below, we can see that our intrepid turtle has to journey through twelve channels over a twenty-four-hour period. It takes two hours to traverse one channel and therefore eight hours to travel through one four-channel set. Naturally, there are three four-channel sets, comprising the twelve channels in total.

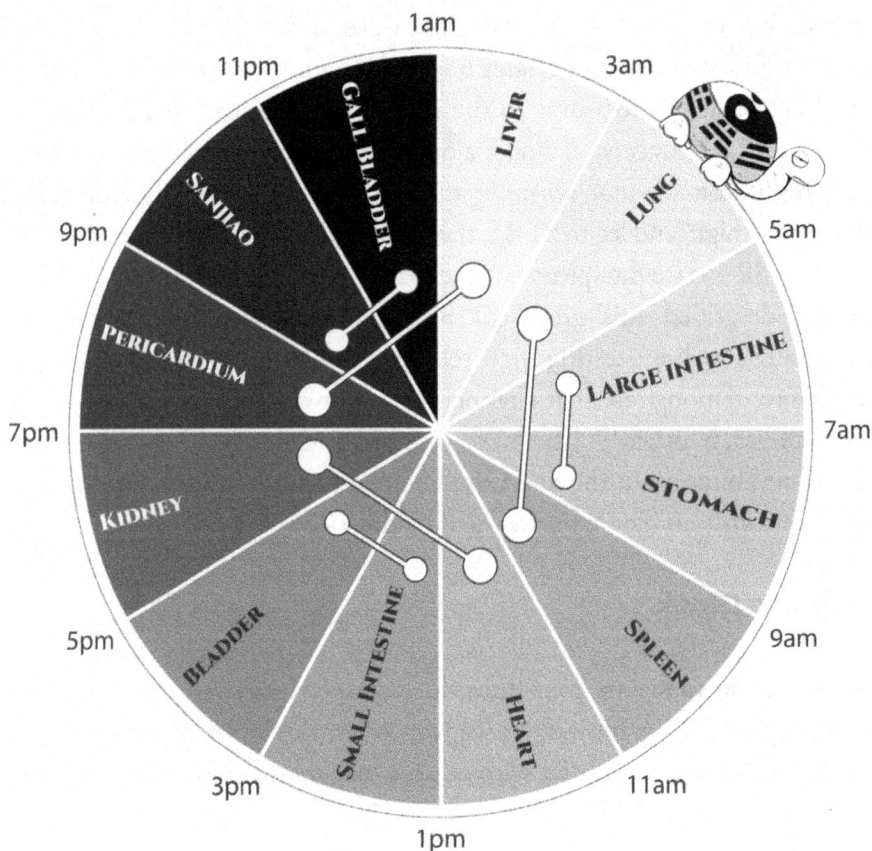

Pairings chart: the long lines link internal-external pairs; the short lines connect the six-channel pairs; the longitudinal axes show *shigo* polar channel pairs

The pairings chart above shows that each of these pairs forms a long axis or pole. Just like the North and South Poles of the earth, each pair forms a longitudinal axis. This relationship is what Dr Tan called clock opposites and what Dr Manaka called polar channel pairs.

Each channel experiences a peak and a trough every twelve hours. If the surge reaches the heart channel between 11:00 a.m. and 1:00 p.m., the energy in the heart channel is strongest at this time. Twelve hours later, however, the surge is as far away as it can be, so the energy in the heart channel is at its lowest, like a slow-moving tsunami pulling the water away from a beach before it eventually surges back.

If we now consider the same times in relation to the gall bladder channel, we can see the same surge phenomenon in reverse. Between 11:00 p.m. and 1:00 a.m., the energy in the gall bladder channel is at its strongest. Conversely, twelve hours later, at lunchtime, when the surge is at its furthest away, the energy in the gall bladder will be at its lowest. So, the Chinese Clock establishes a new set of yin-yang relationships between seemingly unrelated channels. We can see this relationship between heart and gall bladder in the chart below. In the words of former American first lady, Michelle Obama, "When they go low, we go high". This relationship is repeated for each of the six polar pairs, each peaking and troughing twelve hours apart.

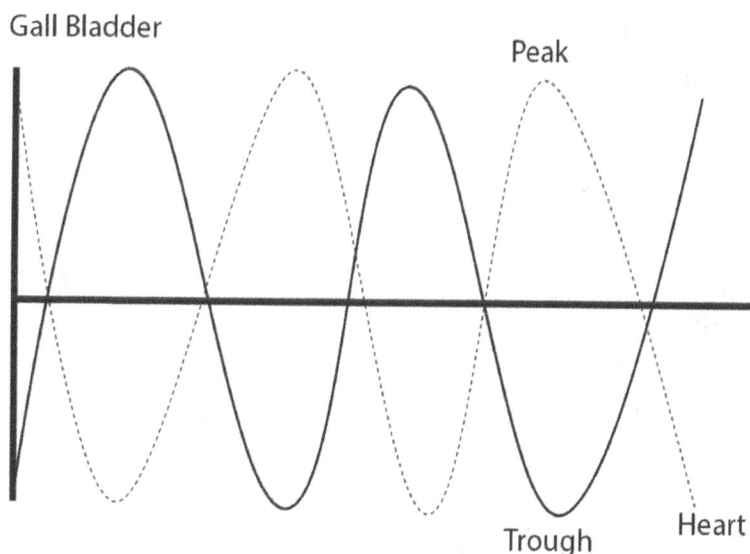

When gall bladder channel goes low, the heart channel goes high!

When we compare the three pairing systems. It is interesting to note that *shigo* contains elements of both the previous two. Internal-external principles pair yin and yang channels, either on the arm or leg. Six-channel theory pairs yang channels on the arm with yang channels on the leg, or yin channels on the arm with yin channels on the leg.

Shigo, by contrast, pairs a yin channel on the arm with a yang channel on the leg, or a yang channel on the arm with a yin channel on the leg. If you also exploit left-right relationships, this can be a very dynamic method.

Many practitioners and styles have exploited this theory. Manaka developed a whole root treatment using polar channel pairs that he integrated into his octahedral model. In Toyohari, *shigo* needling is used for branch treatment. Dr Tan integrated this pairing into his Systems Matrix.

Ontake 1, 2, 3

Now that we have discussed holographic systems and three systems for pairing channels, we can look at how Dr Tan's approach can be adapted for Ontake. Dr Tan described a three-step process which became the title of his book *Acupuncture 1, 2, 3* and inspired the title of this chapter.

Dr Tan's Three Steps

1. Identify the sick channel.
2. Determine the treatment channel based on the five pairing systems.
3. Select points according to the mirroring and imaging formats.[126]

Three Steps for Ontake

When using Ontake for pain relief, these steps can be adapted as follows:
1. Identify the sick channel.
2. Select a balancing channel from the three pairing systems.
3. Select treatment areas according to the mirroring and imaging formats and apply Ontake at the area's frequency.

1) Identify the sick channel.

Dr Tan used the Balance Method to treat all kinds of diseases, both internal and external. In the context of Ontake, we are only treating pain. Identifying the sick channel is therefore much more straightforward: we merely need to know the

---

126   Tan, R. T. (2007). Acupuncture 1, 2, 3. San Diego, CA: R. Tan.

channel pathways and map those onto where the patient feels pain. Sometimes more than one channel will be affected, particularly in conditions like neck and shoulder pain. In these cases, it is worth palpating carefully for reactions, so you can list and prioritise the affected channels.

2) Select a balancing channel from one of the three pairing systems.

When performing a tension assessment, you should already have in mind the three channels that will balance the problem channel. Although a tension assessment provides only general information, you should already have an idea of the sick channel where the patient is feeling pain at the start of treatment. You can focus in on those channels you think may help to balance the pain. Look, stroke, and press for reactions.

3) Select treatment areas according to the mirroring and imaging formats.

Medical acupuncturist Jochen Gleditsch notes that acupuncture points on microacupuncture systems have an on/off switch. When an area is healthy, the related points on the system are switched off, but when an area is sick, the points relating to that area switch on and become tender.[127]

This is actually no different from the Japanese perspective on channel points, which says it is not productive to treat channel points unless you can ascertain that they are, in Toyohari jargon, "currently alive" (i.e., switched on and activated). Denmei Shudo, the foremost exponent of Meridian Therapy states that there must be a reaction at a point before you consider using it. Most moxibustion practitioners in Japan locate a painful point and make that the point for treatment. They would not consider applying *okyu* (small cone moxibustion) on a point unless there is a reaction.[128]

I'm hesitant to attribute an on/off switch to microacupuncture points alone; I would argue that this is a property of all acupuncture points, including channel points. This question becomes even more relevant when we consider that Ontake is too big to treat acupuncture points precisely; it is better suited to broader areas. Can we say that whole *areas* on a hologram are "currently alive"? We have already

127 Hecker, H., Steveling, A., & Peuker, E. (2005). *Microsystems Acupuncture: The Complete Guide: Ear-Scalp-Mouth-Hand.* Stuttgart: Thieme, p. XIII.

128 Mizutani, J. (1988). Practical Moxibustion Therapy. *North American Journal of Oriental Medicine, 6,* p. 16.

seen how the Japanese focus much attention on abnormal tissue findings such as *kyo* and *jitsu*. How can we ascertain that an area of a hologram is switched on and will have a therapeutic effect before we apply Ontake? As usual, the answer is palpation, palpation, palpation!

When choosing treatment areas on the upper or lower limb, the first step is to examine them closely. You may see sunken or swollen areas that get your attention. The next step is palpation. There are several holographic mappings and channel pairings. Let palpation be your guide. The reaction that feels most *kyo* or most *jitsu* is likely to be the most effective.

At this step, instead of needling the treatment channel, we apply Ontake at the frequency of that channel until the reactions are clear (usually less than a minute). Reactions clearing could mean that: a cold area becomes warm, a sunken area develops more lustre, swollen areas change tonus, tenderness fades, or crunchy crystals feel less reactive. Essentially, you are looking for changes from your starting point. With Ontake, this does not take long. Once you sense change, check with the patient on the location of the pain, range of motion or intensity of the pain.

The direction of stimulation should generally flow with the channel, but this is not an absolute rule. The main goal is to balance the *kyo* and *jitsu* of the area being treated and clear the reactions.

Chasing the Pain

When you want to check on the progress or effect of the treatment, it is more useful to check by asking "Where is the pain now?" rather than "How is the pain now?". This is because the pain will often move during treatment. Dr Tan described this process as "chasing the pain". If the pain migrates, you may need to chase it up and down the image with the bamboo, or if it moves laterally, for example from BL to GB, you need to change to a new balancing channel. You may also need to change your bamboo technique. Bamboo is intrinsically mobile, and you can be much more flexible and responsive than with needling.

DU 14 Dazhui

DU 14 is the intersection of all the yang channels. It can therefore be very helpful for symptoms on any yang channel. Rubbing in double time or vibrating work really well. You can "aim" slightly to the left or to the right with the bamboo. I often finish treating pain on a yang channel by vibrating at DU 14 at the appropriate frequency.

Side of Treatment

In TCM treatment, acupuncture is very commonly applied bilaterally. This is not the case in many styles of Japanese acupuncture or the Balance Method, where considerable thought has gone into "getting more bang for your buck" by selecting the best side for treatment. Dr Tan, for example, developed rules for the side of treatment for each of his five pairing systems.

Internal/External and Six-Channel Pairs

For internal/external and six-channel pairs, Dr Tan's default was to treat only on the side opposite to the pain. In my experience, bamboo works well when applied in this way—most of the time. On rare occasions, it is evident through palpation or visual inspection that there are more reactions on the balancing channel on the same side as the pain, and in these cases, it makes more sense to treat ipsilaterally and then check the result.

Dr Tan did not favour treating bilaterally with these two pairings, but Ontake seems more forgiving than needling. Although I prefer to work on one side only, on rare occasions I have used both sides, especially for internal/external pairings.

Shigo

Shigo is a more interesting topic because Dr Tan's principles for the side of treatment are different from those developed for *shigo* in MSA or Toyohari. Dr Tan taught that when using this pairing, we should treat the same side, or, for bilateral problems, treat bilaterally.

In Toyohari, *shigo* is applied for the treatment of acute, painful conditions on the opposite side of the pain. Using the opposite side exploits not only the polarities inherent in the *shigo* relationships, such as yin and yang and hand and foot, but also the polarity of left and right, which makes this a very dynamic treatment option. Manaka also developed a very specific polar channel pair root treatment that, for the most part, uses abdominal palpation to select between left and right treatment areas, as well as between the other oppositions of his octahedral model: front/back and upper/lower.

Thus, there are clear differences in approach between Japanese styles and Dr Tan's style that need to be taken into consideration when applying Ontake with this pairing. My clinical experience with *shigo* and these systems and styles leads me to conclude that in the context of each system, those rules are appropriate. Whilst I love doing *shigo* needling with a gold needle on the opposite side of the body in Toyohari, this default rule does not work so well in MSA or the Balance Method. Dr Tan's selection of the side of treatment involves stimulating an acupuncture microsystem superimposed over the channel system, and using this model, I have found it more effective to follow his rules. Thus, for the Ontake treatment of pain with *shigo*, I recommend using the same side or performing treatment bilaterally as the default.

I do make exceptions to this based on palpation. If there are very clear reactions on one side, it makes sense to treat them. Japanese acupuncture is very pragmatic, and pragmatism often trumps theory. As you get more experienced, palpation may give you better results for determining the side of treatment than rules.

Examples

In the examples below, there is an important distinction to make between conventional needling and Ontake treatment. Needling treats points. Ontake is a regional moxibustion treatment that covers broad lines or areas. The aim of Ontake treatment is to balance *kyo* and *jitsu* in a region or line. Thus, Ontake treatment extends beyond the point selections of Tan balancing and treats lines along the hologram.

Neck pain is very common in clinic. Let's look at neck pain on the bladder channel on the left. If the bladder channel is the sick channel, then we should check the balancing channels: the kidney, small intestine, and lung.

Using the reverse image, the "glove puppet" (described earlier), then we can see that the hand or foot treats the head, and the wrist and ankle joints treat the neck and neck joint. Thus, we can look for reactions on the image of the head to the neck from around KID 3 to KID 9, SI 6 to SI 7, and LU 6 to LU 9. Let us imagine that we found reactions and indurations on the lung channel, perhaps with hollowness around LU 7 and indurations at LU 6. Then we should apply bamboo along the arm at 126 beats per minute. This might include rolling all the way between LU 10 and LU 5 to balance the *kyo* and *jitsu* of the channel.

Headache is also very common in clinic. Sometimes people arrive with one. In the case of temporal headache on the gall bladder channel, the balancing channels will be the liver, triple burner, and heart. Using the reverse image (the glove puppet), look for reactions from LIV 1 to LIV 5, TB 1 to TB 5, and HT 4 to HT 9.

Using the normal image, you can also check out HT 1 to HT 3 or TB 10 to TB 15. This is an example where bamboo can achieve marvellous results for a problem with a surprising choice of points. Of course, relieving headache by rolling on the LIV 3 area (108) can be explained by the known indications for LIV 3 without talking about the reverse image, but treating headache by rolling warm bamboo at HT 1 through HT 3 on the same side is more challenging to explain by classical theory.

There are no indications in the traditional literature that HT 1 is a point for treating temporal headaches. In the normal image, the top of the shoulder relates to the top of the head. As HT 1 is in the shoulder, it should affect the head. The heart channel is paired to the gall bladder channel through *shigo*, so treating the heart channel ipsilaterally relieves temporal headache.

This model also sheds light on more famous points with indications for the head— LU 7, the main point for the head and neck, for example. The lung channel is the polar opposite of the bladder channel, which flows through the back of the neck. Its location on the hologram places it just below the occiput.

Another example is LI 4, the main point for the face and mouth. It pairs with the stomach channel through the six-channel system, and its location on the hologram is on the hand in the reverse image, corresponding to the lower part of the head. These correlations reinforce ideas from classical acupuncture.

Cases

As we have seen, bamboo should be applied as a branch treatment following root treatment. In most of the examples below, bamboo was given after root treatment either with Toyohari or MSA methods. In some cases, where the pain was severe, it was applied before the root treatment.

Female: 30. Temporal Headaches on the Left and Right.

This athletic young woman was trying to conceive, but she had very irregular periods. It turned out she liked to run marathons. She was diagnosed as a liver-deficient type. On this occasion, she arrived with a temporal headache on both sides. On a one to ten scale, the pain on the right was a seven in severity. On the left, five out of ten.

The gall bladder was diagnosed as the sick channel. In the reverse image (glove puppet), the hand mirrors the head. The heart channel is the polar channel pair of the gall bladder channel. When Ontake was rolled on the left at HT 7 to HT 9 (126) the pain reduced to zero on the left and to three on the right. Ontake was then applied to HT 7 to HT 9 on the right for thirty seconds, until she reported the pain gone. In this case, rolling the *shigo* channel on the left cleared the symptoms on the left, also reducing symptoms on the right.

Female: 30. Scleroderma.

This woman looked like she had been in a fire. Her skin was thick and leathery all over her face, arms, and legs, and she could not open her hands. She had joint pain everywhere. The pain in her finger joints was severe. Her left-hand pain was a seven out of ten in severity, and her right was four out of ten.

The skin on the dorsum of both hands was very badly affected, and although the yin channels were clearly in contracture, treatment was aimed at the three arm yang channels. Her right foot was colder, and the tendons more pronounced than on the left, indicating a deficiency. Ontake was applied using the normal mirror on the right foot to treat LIV 1 to LIV 3, ST 43 to ST 45, and GB 41 to GB 44. The liver pairs with the small intestine (*shigo*), the stomach with the large intestine (six channels), and the gall bladder with the triple burner (six channels). These channels were selected partly because of their pairings and partly because they are all on the dorsum of the foot, meaning they could all be treated at the same time. These points were rolled lightly for thirty seconds, resulting in a marked drop in pain. Rolling was then continued for five minutes, much longer than usual with bamboo, until the patient reported the pain was at zero in both hands.

Here we can see, once again, that only treating one side affected both sides.

Female: 36. Pregnant with Back Pain.

This woman was thirty-five weeks pregnant and had developed pain on the right from BL 18 outwards (inner and outer bladder line). There were reactions on the right lung channel (polar channel pair).

In the reverse image, the forearm corresponds to the upper back. Bamboo was applied from LU 5 to LU 7 (126). After thirty seconds, the pain migrated to below the scapula (small intestine). Using the reverse image and polar channel pairing on the opposite leg, bamboo was applied to LIV 5 to LIV 8. The pain reduced. The same area was treated on the right, and the pain disappeared.

Conclusion

Dr Tan simplified, codified, and popularised a very effective system of acupuncture by combining two different treatment modalities: balancing pairs of channels through various pairing systems while employing holographic mappings to choose the area to be needled. Interestingly, Dr Manaka himself used the same juxtaposition of systems, using another holographic system, the Hirata zones, to focus his point selection for treating pancreatitis with ion-pumping cords.

Tan's Balance Method is far more complex and multi-layered than the simple explanation in this chapter, and he used many more holograms than those described above. The work in this chapter is not an attempt to redefine the Balance Method. Instead, my goal was to add the perspective of the Balance Method to moxibustion, expanding the range of possibilities for Ontake treatment.

It is the contrast between the effects of needling and moxibustion that makes this adaptation interesting to consider. Bamboo has two areas of physical effect. It generates heat, both radiant and direct, which feels soothing and helps the muscles relax very quickly. Secondly, it affects the soft tissue both by compression or stretching, as with simple rolling techniques, and with percussion, such as with knocking or tapping. These percussive and rhythmic strokes acquire even more healing momentum when applied with a metronome at the appropriate frequency of the meridian.

This is something new, very different from any other moxibustion technique and different again from the retained needling and deep insertion of the Balance Method. What is more, it is easy to adjust the treatment with bamboo, chasing the pain in real-time by minutely changing the trajectory of the strokes—far easier than changing needle locations.

In conclusion, importing Tan's Balance Method theory into bamboo treatment adds new dimensions to both. On the one hand, it liberates us from needling. On the other, it focuses Ontake for very specific and dynamic applications. It is perhaps for these reasons that pain relief with bamboo can be so effective.

Summary

Holographic systems exist all over the body from the very small, such as the ear or philtrum, to the very large, such as Dr Tan's normal and reverse images on the arm and leg. Dr Tan's system combines traditional channel pairings with holographic systems, and it is this combining of systems gives his method its dynamic effect.

Ontake 1, 2, 3 adapts Dr Tan's three steps, adding one more layer: the meridian frequency of the treatment channel. The default rules for side of treatment can be overridden by palpatory findings.

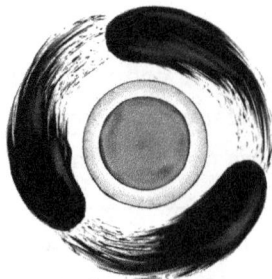

CHAPTER 12

BALANCING THE OCTAHEDRON

Applying Ontake to Manaka's octahedral model, opposite regions of the body, and channel pairings can create dynamic and surprising effects.

Disorders manifesting symptoms on the posterior aspect of the body are often most effectively treated on the anterior aspect of the body, and vice versa. Lumbago back pain, for example, can be treated by stimulating the sensitive points of the thorax and abdomen. ... In accordance with this "principle of opposites", one should also treat complaints of the upper body by points on the lower body, and vice versa.

—Yoshio Manaka[129]

---

129 Manaka, Y., & Urquhart, I. (1972). *The Layman's Guide to Acupuncture*. New York: Weatherhill, p. 121.

Re-Presenting the Octahedral Model

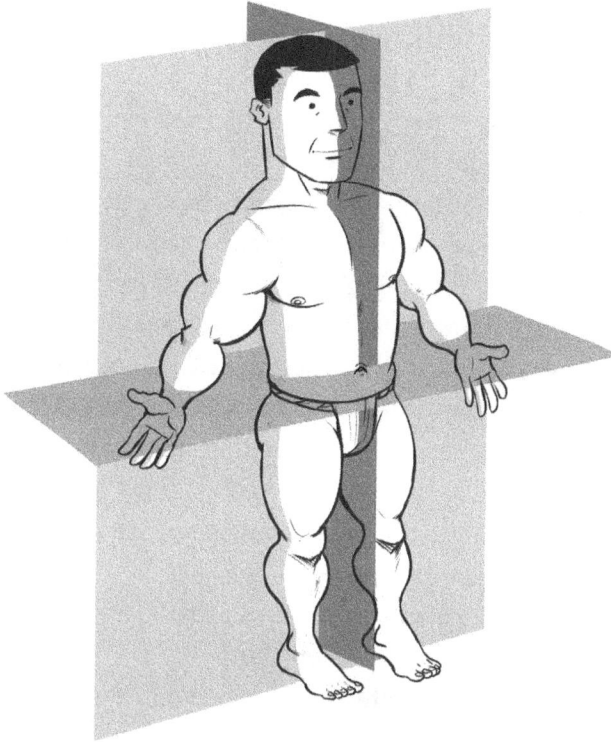

The three axes of the body create four anterior and four posterior quadrants.

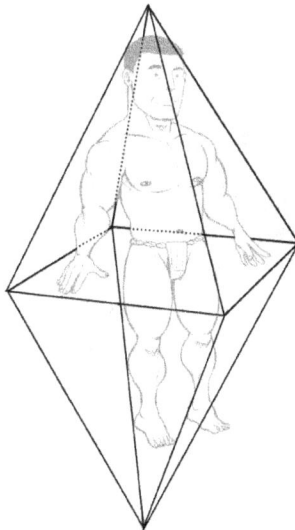

Manaka's octahedral model developed a root treatment
adjusting the flow of qi in the octants of the body.

Manaka's octahedral model theory starts with the most basic of assumptions in anatomy: that there are three axes in the body. One axis separates right from left, another front from back, and another top from bottom. These axes give us a three-dimensional way to map the body, such as left, right; anterior, posterior; and superior, inferior. Manaka noticed that if you draw the axes in and then connect the ends, they make a geometric shape: an octahedron. Manaka had read Buckminster Fuller extensively, who observed that the octahedron is the most stable shape in geometry.

An octahedron is an eight-sided figure, but in classical acupuncture anatomy (i.e., the structure of the meridian system), the channels are organised in sets of twelve. There are twelve cutaneous regions, twelve collateral channels, twelve sinew channels, twelve primary channels, and twelve divergent channels. There is only one set of vessels, of which there are eight. These are the *Kikei Hachi Miyaku*, the Eight Extraordinary Vessels, and it was these eight vessels that drew Manaka's attention.

Could the Eight Extras, in some way, relate to the octahedron enfolded within the three axes of the body? This hypothesis was explored in great detail in *Chasing the Dragon's Tail*, a landmark acupuncture textbook that explores and tests many assumptions of acupuncture with a scientific eye.

For this chapter, we can map out Manaka's octahedron on the torso in a very simple way. The Ren Mai and Du Mai run along the anterior and posterior midline dividing the body into left and right halves. The Dai Mai runs horizontally along the abdomen at the umbilicus, extending posteriorly to L 2, giving us upper and lower halves. The anterior and posterior halves of the body are defined by the Yang Wei Mai, running along the median line of the lateral torso.[130] Manaka considered the master and coupled points P 6, TB 5, SP 4, and GB 41 to create similar median dividing lines on the limbs.

Returning to the ideas about yin and yang touched on in chapter 3, when we consider yin and yang in clinical terms, we look for relationships that are either harmonised or out of balance. We can imagine a see-saw with two kids sitting on it. If the kids are of equal weight, the see-saw is level. Put a heavier kid on one end and a lighter one on the other, and you see an imbalance. One side goes up, and one side goes down. This is one way of representing the relative amounts of yin and yang in the body. TCM textbooks also represent these shifting balances with a series of column graphs.[131] In all models, to treat a problem, we need to rectify an imbalance of yin and yang.

---

130 Matsumoto, K., & Birch, S. (1986). *Extraordinary Vessels*. Brookline: Paradigm Publications.

131 Maciocia, G. (1989). *The Foundations of Chinese Medicine: A Comprehensive Text for Acupuncturists and Herbalists*. Edinburgh: Churchill Livingstone, p. 13.

The most important thing to consider when using Manaka's octahedral model with Ontake is that the eight facets are in dynamic equilibrium. This is like having four see-saws, all chained and linked and moving in interlinked relationships. Upper balances lower, left balances right, front balances back, and vice versa.

When teaching, Dr Manaka "often used a complex mobile to illustrate the multidimensionality of clinical reality".[132] Similarly, Stephen Birch has sometimes used model octahedrons made out of coat hanger wire or small magnets to illustrate the structural distortions that can take place throughout the model when applying pressure onto one of its eight facets.

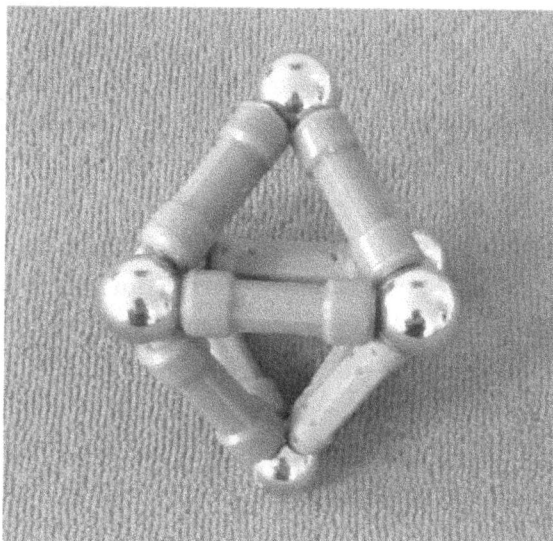

Magnetic octahedron (photo by Marian Fixler).

Dr Manaka considered the flow of qi in the channels in the eight octants of the body to be a key to rectifying the condition of the body and curing disease. All of this sounds complicated, and indeed, Manaka's thoughts about the octahedron and what he called the X-signal system drew on vast reams of scientific research. Clinical applications with Ontake are far less complicated than the theory. We will now look at practical ways to use Manaka's octants when treating pain.

132   Birch, S., & Felt, R. (1999). *Understanding Acupuncture*. Edinburgh: Churchill Livingstone, p. 139.

From Theory to Practice

If we divide the torso into four anterior quadrants and four posterior quadrants, we can label them as follows: anterior upper right (AUR), anterior upper left (AUL), anterior lower right (ALR), anterior lower left (ALL), posterior upper right (PUR), posterior upper left (PUL), posterior lower right (PLR), and posterior lower left (PLL).

Like Dr Tan, Manaka was also very concerned with balancing within his model of treatment, and he brought to bear all the principles of yin and yang, lower and upper, front and back, and left and right to balance his octahedron using many different methods and modalities.

For the application of Ontake, this becomes very simple: all we need to consider is that upper balances lower, left balances right, front balances back, and vice versa. These principles are not unique to Manaka and are common currency in many styles of acupuncture, going back to the *Nei Jing*.

These ideas, together with the simplicity of applying Ontake, have led to the development of a different routine for selecting acupuncture points and areas to treat, this time according to balancing quadrants. Sometimes this literally means tapping on a whole quadrant or pair of quadrants to release an opposite area. At other times, this means choosing paired channels on opposite quadrants. When the dynamic effects of the points and channels used in this way are compared with their traditional indications, treating with Ontake has produced surprising results.

Quadrants 1, 2, 3

With another hats-off to Dr Tan, this Ontake routine follows another three-step protocol, mostly using the same three pairing systems from the previous chapter (internal/external, six channels, and *shigo*). Sometimes no pairings are used at all, with tapping on the broad expanse of the entire quadrant providing sufficient results. When doing this, the generic frequencies discussed in chapter 4 are appropriate.

1. Identify the affected quadrant.
2. Choose the opposite quadrant using the three axes of the body.
3. Check the overall lustre of this quadrant. Look for reactions along the paired channels that flow there, according to the pairings above.

Thus, if a problem manifests in the LLQ, at the back, it makes sense to look for and treat reactions in the URQ, on the front. In practice, there are fewer pairings to consider, because not all the channels in these three pairing systems will flow through the opposite quadrant.

As an example, let us consider sacral and buttock pain on the left. This is in the PLL quadrant, affecting either bladder or gall bladder. Thus, we should examine the lustre and tone of the AUR quadrant, focusing in particular on the kidney or lung (pairing with bladder) and the heart (pairing with gall bladder).

This system works particularly well for problems on the torso, although quadrant theory does include the upper and lower limbs. In my practice, however, I prefer to apply this system more for pain relief on the torso, because Dr Tan's mirrors work so well on the arm and leg.

The diagrams below show the balancing relationships between the quadrants.

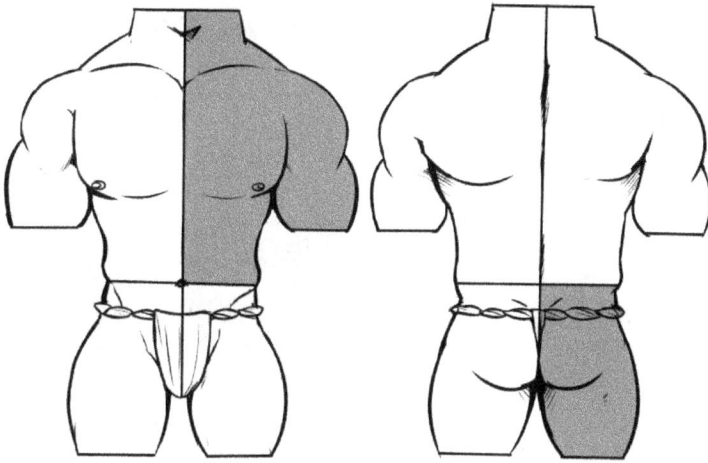

1. AUL/PLR.

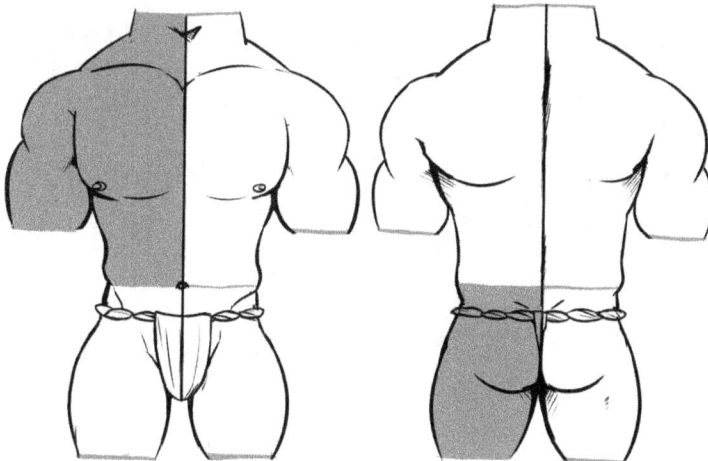

2. AUR/PLL.

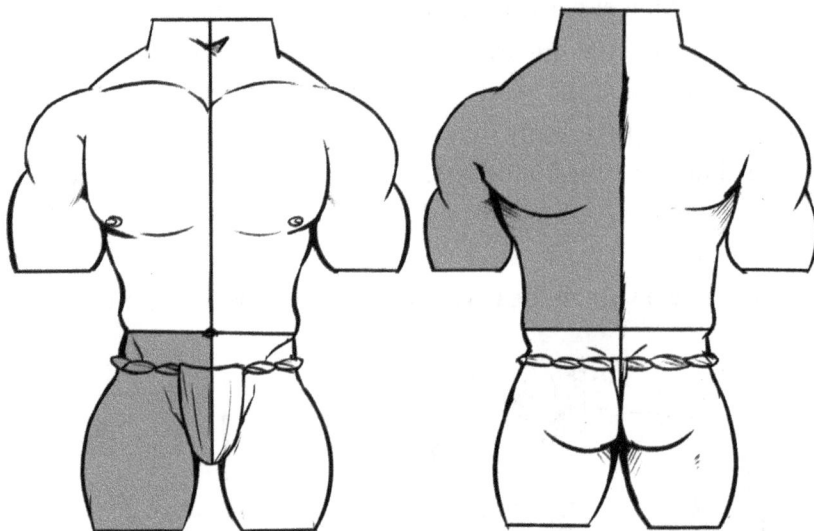

3. ALR/PUL.

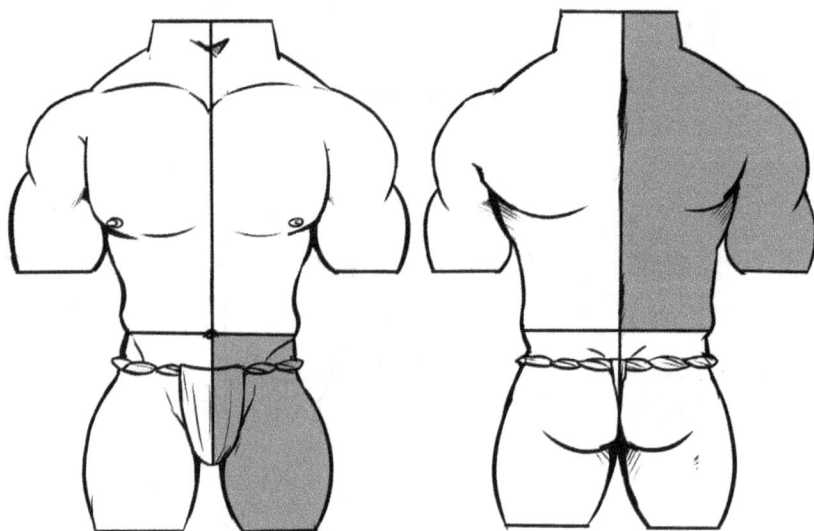

4. ALL/PUR.

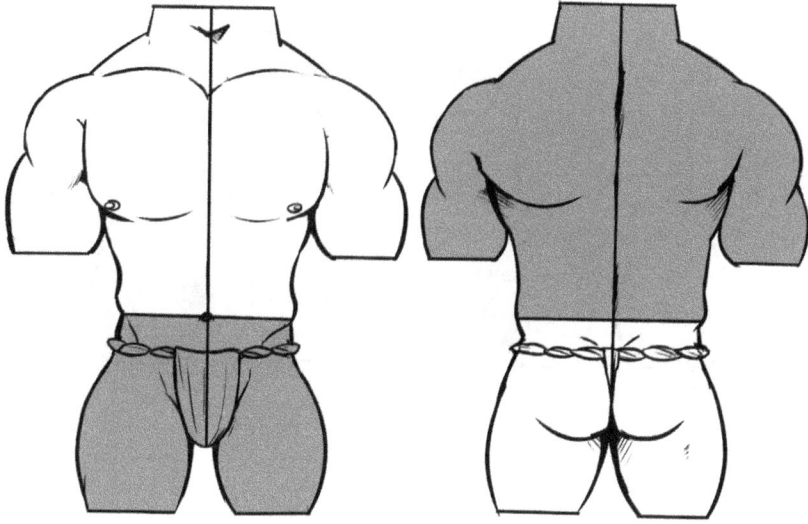

5. ALL + ALR / PUR + PUL.

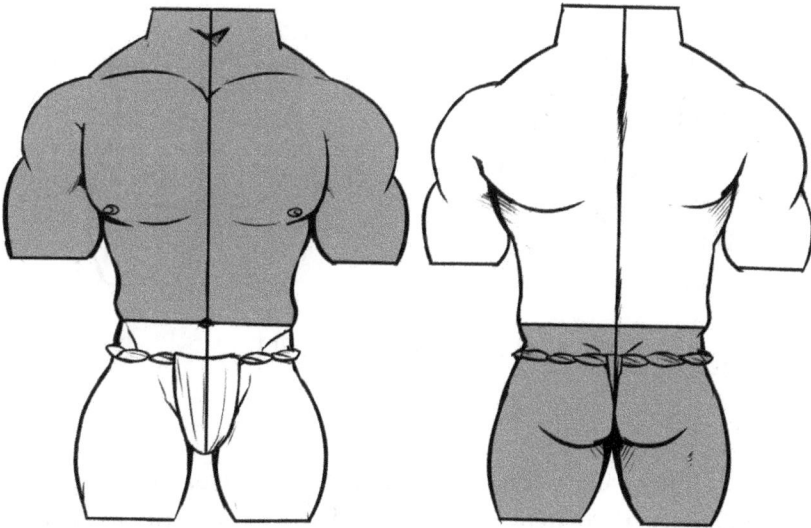

6. AUL + AUR / PLR + PLL.

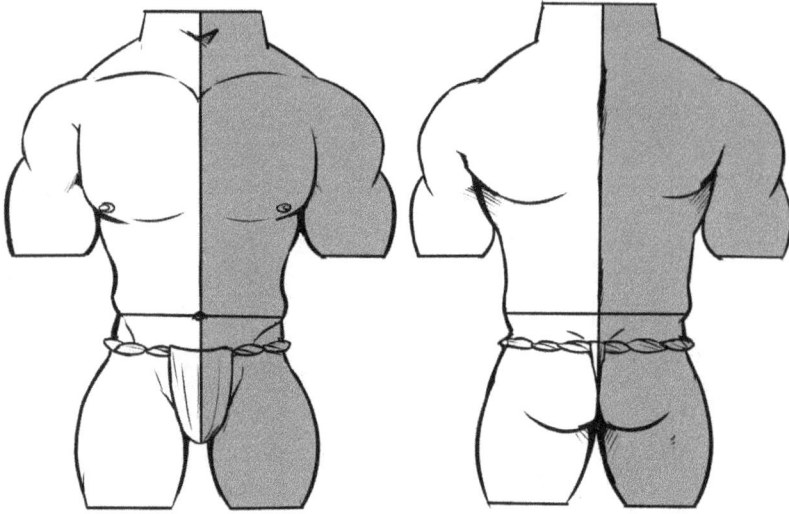

7. AUL + ALL / PLR + PUR.

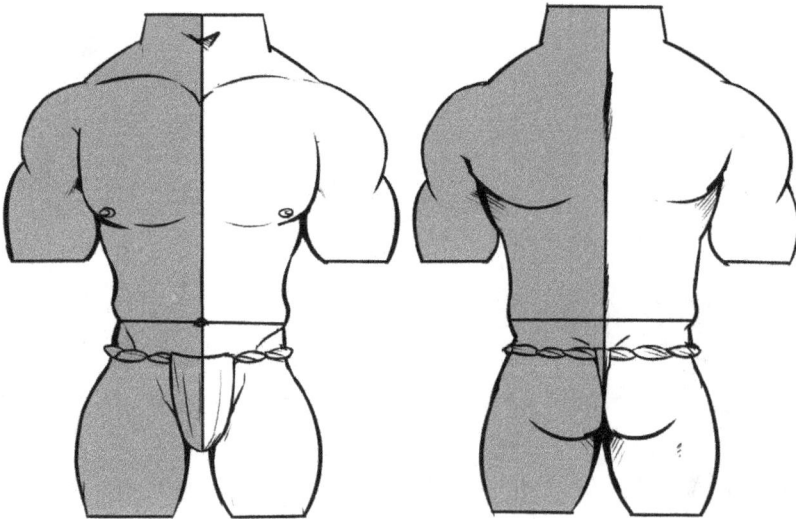

8. ALR + AUR / PUL + PLL.

Occasionally, the pain is on the midline, or perhaps slightly lateral to the midline, in which case there may be little or no left-right polarity to exploit. In these cases, apply bamboo on the corresponding opposite quadrant as usual, but on the midline. If the pain is slightly lateral, then tap slightly lateral to the midline on the opposite side.

Cases

Elderly Male: Secondary Bone Cancer.

This frail old man was feeling tremendous pain in the left iliosacral joint, and he had sciatic pain going down his left leg. The pain was in the bladder channel in the posterior lower left quadrant (PLL). If we use the rules of opposites, the balancing quadrant is anterior upper right (AUR). If we use the same rules for choosing balancing channels as in Dr Tan's system described in the previous chapter, the paired channels for bladder in this area are the kidney or lung, as the small intestine does not flow through the anterior quadrant.

The right LU 1, LU 2 and KID 27 area was very dry and deficient, which required tapping, then touching and closing at the lung and kidney channel frequencies (126 and 120). Previously unable to straighten his leg, the patient started to feel relief from the pain within a few seconds and was asleep within a few minutes. Branch treatment of this kind was given first, followed by root treatment when he was feeling comfortable. Each treatment gave great palliative pain relief that lasted several days.

This patient was my first to be treated with Ontake by balancing quadrants on the front and back, upper and lower, and left and right. The concept has since proved to work in many clinical situations, especially when the pain is on the torso.

Female: Late 30s. Sore Throat.

Ontake was applied on the abdomen, specifically on the kidney, stomach, and spleen channels (120,132, and 132, respectively). This gave some relief simply by balancing upper and lower points. Perhaps this moderate response was because we were only using one polarity, balancing anterior upper quadrants with anterior lower quadrants. Merely using the polarity of upper and lower, there was not enough differential to cause a big shift. With the patient sitting up, tapping was applied to the spine from L-2 to S-4 (104). Then deeper rolling was applied. With the additional polarity of front and back, the sore throat cleared up immediately.

Female: 27. Sore Throat.

She had been working too hard and was stressed. Moxa on LU 10 and root treatment relieved some of the pain but not all. The pain was slightly worse on the left than the right. Reactions were found on either side of the spine, just above the sacrum from L-1 to L-5/S-1. Tapping and rolling were applied with bamboo on the midline (104) and bladder (112), with more emphasis on the right side. The sore throat was fully relieved in less than a minute.

Treating the sacrum area has become my go-to treatment for sore throat. Once when teaching in Japan, my demonstration model had a sore throat. As there were fifty other participants, I was reluctant to expose her sacrum to such a large group. This time I treated through her trousers, allowing the heat to penetrate, changing sides as the pain shifted in her throat. Her pain had been quite severe, a seven out of ten, and by the end of what felt like a long five minutes of demonstration, it had reduced to three out of ten.

In my mind, this was slightly disappointing, as I was trying to present the efficacy of Ontake with sore throats, and until then, I had had an unbroken record of complete success. I put the slow result down to working through her clothes, which meant she did not easily feel the heat. Thirty minutes later, she approached me in the tea break to say the soreness had completely gone. I should have been more understanding of the process. The reduced dosage had simply taken longer to trigger the changes.

Nevertheless, I still marvel at how Ontake can demonstrate and utilise these core beliefs in TEAM theory. The lower part really does balance the upper. The back really does balance the front. We will look at this simple idea more in the discussion of *kubi koshi*.

Female: 30. Upper Back Pain.

She had chronic upper back pain and arrived with a stiff upper back that was tight on both sides. The upper back comprises both posterior upper quadrants. Her abdomen felt very cold, so bamboo was applied at stomach frequency, simply to warm the abdomen, which is anterior and inferior. There was no attempt to find channel pairings. Tapping, touching and closing, and very light rolling techniques were applied until her tummy felt evenly warm. At this point, her back pain released completely. No channel pairing was necessary, as warming the abdomen (lower anterior quadrants) freed the upper back (upper posterior quadrants).

This case is very interesting. There are no indications for upper back pain in the points on the abdomen. When teaching, Stephen Birch has made the point that he can "make up a story" to answer a question and explain why something is happening. By this he means that there is no way of knowing the mechanism, but we can have a go at postulating something.

We can certainly create a narrative that using lower Ren points such as REN 4 could warm the abdomen and pull down counterflow qi from the head, but this misses the point here. The body's octahedral balancing mechanisms are very simple. If the upper back is tight and the tummy is cold, warm the tummy!

Female: 30. Mid-Back Pain.

This woman had mid-back pain on either side of the spine from T-9 to T-12. Simple tapping was applied along the kidney channel from KID 16 to KID 21 (120). The pain improved right away, but it seemed to move down to the lower part of the spine. To chase the pain, tapping was continued, followed by pressing with the lip of the bamboo higher up on the chest on the kidney channel, just below the bra line. At this point, the pain disappeared.

The same patient came back a few months later with central back pain in the spine between T-7 and T-10. Ontake was applied to the anterior midline from REN 15 to REN 12 (104). While tapping lightly for a mere four bars (sixteen beats), the pain reduced then disappeared.

Once again, we can see that quadrant balancing is very simple and uses points that have no traditional indications for back pain. In terms of quadrants, however, these points make more sense. The Du channel goes through the posterior midline and is flanked on either side by the bladder channel. The Ren channel goes through the anterior midline and is flanked on either side by the kidney channel. Seen like this, it makes complete sense that supplementing these kidney points could treat tension in the back.

If yin and yang balance each other, then exploiting opposite polarities of yin and yang, upper and lower, left and right, and front and back should be high on our list of priorities when choosing points and channels. Even at its simplest, Manaka's octahedral model is simply a useful filter to help you find and exploit these polarities, focusing your palpation and enabling you to zone in more quickly to those areas that need treating.

Naso Muno and *Kubi Koshi*

Playing with Manaka's octahedral model in these ways triggered me to experiment with other vertical relationships in the body. Before exploring these thoughts, we should first digress to an important concept in Toyohari, known as *naso muno*.

Naso Muno

The Toyohari Association of Japan bases its approach to acupuncture on the Five Element Meridian Therapy model (*Keiraku Chiryo*). Toyohari, however, was an association initially set up by and for blind practitioners, although in later years they opened their doors first to sighted practitioners and then to practitioners from overseas. Without that change of policy, this book would never have been written! These origins, and the continuing majority membership of blind practitioners, have led to the evolution, even by Japanese standards, of a very palpation-based acupuncture style, as well as some unique clinical methods and approaches.

Naso muno treatment is a specialisation in Toyohari. Both the ST 12 and ST 30 areas are said to be rich in connections to other channels: ST 12 is where all the yang channels meet (except the bladder) and is thought to be where the yang channels of the leg go deep. ST 30 is said to be where they surface.[133] However, these rich connections have not led to many clinical uses for the points. Chinese textbooks are quite terse when it comes to indications for ST 12 (mostly cough), and needling it is also considered a little risky because of its proximity to the upper lobe of the lungs.

Kodo Fukushima, the founder of the Toyohari Association, started palpating these areas and the structures close by, and together with other blind colleagues, he gradually developed a sophisticated scale to assess and treat the reactions they found. These reactions ranged from lightly palpated puffiness to deeper, rubbery reactions to muscles that felt hard and unyielding. Along with needling into these reactions, they used their signature non-insertive needle technique, called *sesshokushin* (touch needling). This approach fell somewhere between root treatment and branch treatment and was known simply as supportive treatment.

The *naso* area came to be defined as ST 12 and all of the neck and supraclavicular fossa, extending to the back of the neck. The *muno* area included ST 30 and the ASIS and inguinal grooves, as well as the sacrum and buttocks. Treating reactions in the *naso* area is useful for any kind of dysfunction from the head to the navel. Treating reactions in the *muno area* is useful for any kind of dysfunction below the navel. For example, *naso* treatment can supplement the treatment of anything from headache to insomnia to arthritis in the fingers. *Muno* treatment can supplement the treatment of anything from back pain to infertility to cold feet.

133   Deadman, P., Al-Khafaji, M., & Baker, K. (1998). *A Manual of Acupuncture*. East Sussex, England: Journal of Chinese Medicine Publications.

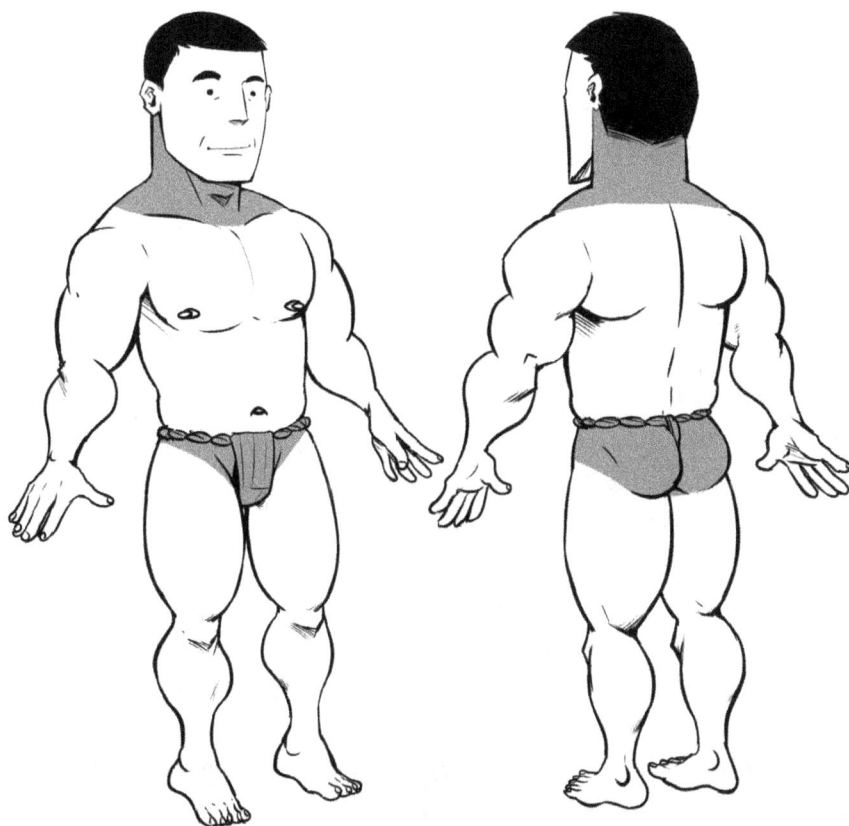

The Toyohari theory of *naso muno* extends the areas influenced by ST 12 and ST 30 into specialised treatment regions at the neck and waist.

Naso muno deploys very specialised treatments that require a high degree of palpatory sensitivity and discrimination, as well as great finesse with conventional needling and *sesshokushin* (touch needling). This brings us to another use for Ontake, which we already encountered briefly during the Bamboo Max whole-body routine.

Ontake lends itself to treating these areas without requiring the same high levels of palpatory or needling skill. Simply rolling the lateral aspect of the neck at 120 beats per minute feels very relaxing and has systemic effects on problems in the upper limb and chest. As ST 12 is an intersection point, you can tap at various yang channel frequencies to affect anywhere on the yang channel network. It is interesting to note that tapping ST 12 at the bladder frequency still has effects on the bladder channel, implying at least a possibility that, counter to classical theory, the bladder channel does, in some way, interact with this point.

At ST 30 and the inguinal region, tapping primarily at 132 beats per minute seems sufficient to release reactions and cause systemic structural shifts, particularly those affecting the uterus, lower back, hip, knees, and feet. This area is also the

Manaka *mu* point for the gall bladder, which may explain why 120 beats per minute also works well.

In Toyohari *naso muno* treatment is applied after root treatment and before branch treatment. In Ontake, it makes sense to palpate the neck or waist during root treatment and try and iron out any reactions at this stage.

The *Kubi Koshi Hypothesis*

In Japanese, *kubi* means "neck", and *koshi* means "waist". Working in the clinic with quadrant theory and *naso muno* requires frequent palpation and assessment and reassessment of the changes taking place during the treatment. Over the past few years, my assistants, Koki Takemoto and Ryo Izawa, and I have started to observe connections between the *naso* and *muno* areas not discussed in the Toyohari literature.

With the patient lying prone, we palpated the sides of the neck, looking for reactions such as swelling and tightness. Where these were present, we also noticed distinct bands of tightness at the sides of the hip in a line upwards from GB 26. Where the tension on the neck was more at the back, we also noticed areas of puffiness around the sacrum and on the lower bladder line. By tapping on these lower areas at the appropriate frequencies, we were repeatedly able to observe significant reductions in the tension in the neck and the alleviation of symptoms in both the neck and the upper limb.

We have seen with holographic theory that each part of the whole reflects and encodes the information of the whole. As this process continued, we noticed more connections; for example, that rolling on the sacrum could relieve sore throat. It seemed that we were slowly uncovering another mirroring hologram. This process has felt like archaeology, with us slowly excavating layers in the fascia to see how the body connects and interacts. What we have pieced together so far is this:

- Rolling on the sacrum consistently relieves sore throat (104).
- Rolling on the coccyx may sometimes affect sensations in the tongue (104).
- Rolling on the sides of the sacrum affects the neck, both anteriorly and posteriorly (112).
- Rolling on the sides of the waist, from GB 26 to lower margin of the ribs (120) softens the sides of the neck, sometimes releasing the opposite side.
- Tapping on the kidney channel below the navel relieves posterior neck reactions (120).
- Tapping on the lower Ren points relieves midline stiffness in the neck (104).
- Tapping on kidney points on the epigastrium relieves mid-back stiffness on the bladder channel (120).

- Tapping on kidney points below the clavicle relieves lower back pain on the bladder channel (120).

These observations combine assumptions about quadrant relationships with ideas from *naso muno*. In a very simplistic way, we can say that the *naso* and *muno* areas reflect each other, but the clinical observations above seem more complex than that, particularly concerning left-right and front-back polarities. Is there a mirroring between the way the cranium sits on the cervical spine and the way the pelvis connects to the lumbar spine?

To answer this, imagine your patient lying in prone position. If you placed a mirror on her mid-back, with the reflecting side facing her head, you would see her actual head and upper torso as well as a reflected image, both joined at the mirror. Now imagine that the reflected head and torso were no longer in prone position but in supine. This gives us an image for the *kubi koshi* hypothesis.

According to this model, we can extrapolate that the kidney and Ren Mai points, from REN 8 at the navel to REN 2 at the pubic symphysis, reflect the Du Mai and the bladder points on the back of the neck from C-7 to the occiput. This would make the whole waist and pelvis area an upside-down mirror of the neck and inferior aspect of the cranium, and REN 8 would be a subtle mirror of DU 14.

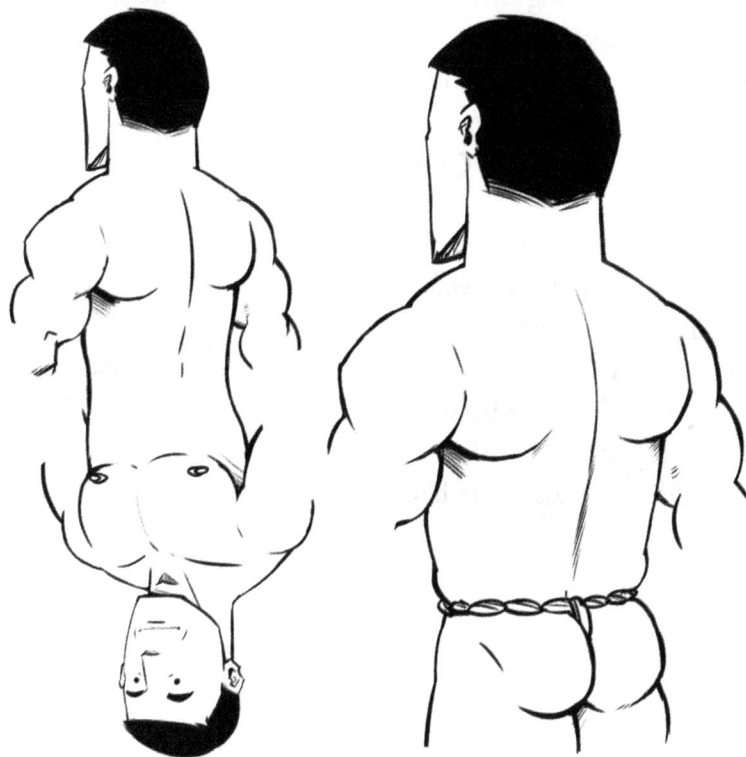

Hypothetical *kubi koshi* hologram.

There is one precedent for this in the Japanese literature: the Hirata zones. In these, the region from the level of T-3 to the occiput is a reverse mirror hologram of the body, and the torso region itself is a normal mirror. It then makes sense that there should be some dynamic correlation between the lower back and the upper neck (see chapter 13).

Testing *Kubi Koshi*

As I write about *kubi koshi*, I'm reminded of Manaka's catchphrase, "Don't believe a word I say!" *Kubi koshi* reactions are quite easy to replicate, and you can test them with ease on your next patient.

1. With a model lying prone, stand at the top of the head and palpate the sides of the neck. You may notice left-right differences between the lateral aspects. In particular, focus on hardness or tightness. Is one side tighter than the other? What is the underlying quality of the neck's lateral muscles? You may find both *kyo* and *jitsu*.
2. Palpate along the lateral waist from the costal margin to the top of the iliac crest. There may be bands of tension lying superficially or deeply along this lateral aspect.
3. Apply Ontake along these tight bands (120) on one side until they loosen up. Then recheck the neck.
4. Repeat on the other side and check the neck again.

Conclusion

Treating the waist in this way is a useful way to address problems in the neck and head. A good time to introduce *kubi koshi* is during the second part of the routine tension assessment, when the patient is lying prone. Take a minute or two to palpate the neck and waist and look for abnormal tissues that mirror each other in some way.

Over time, *kubi koshi* has become an important part of the Ontake repertoire, particularly when palpation of the neck reveals regions where the muscle feels very hard and unyielding, almost bone-like, a sign in Toyohari that a problem is chronic and hard to treat.

Summary

In this chapter, we learned Manaka's complicated octahedral model can be reduced to eight simple tapping zones, four anterior quadrants, and four posterior quadrants. As Ontake is used to treat lines and areas more than points, symptoms in one quadrant can be treated by warming the skin in the opposite quadrant.

Naso muno is a specialised treatment of the neck and waist that originated from the interesting theoretical energetics of two points: ST 12 and ST 30. *Kubi koshi* combines ideas from *naso muno* with quadrant theory to uncover interesting new relationships between the neck and waist. These can be exploited with Ontake.

PART 4

BAMBOO SHOOTS

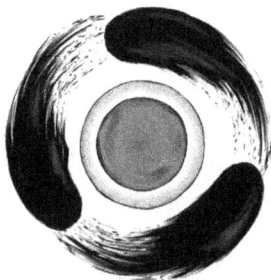

CHAPTER 13

INTEGRATING ONTAKE WITH MANAKA'S FOUR-STEP PROTOCOL

Presenting ways to integrate Ontake into each step of Manaka's four-step protocol (written specifically for practitioners of Manaka-style acupuncture).

Introducing the Hirata zones, useful for practitioners still learning about MSA.

Manaka-Style Acupuncture (MSA)— The Four-Step Protocol

Although Dr Manaka died in 1989, MSA has not stood still. With practitioners in Europe, the Americas, Australia, and Asia, especially in Indonesia, his ideas are widely used, either on their own as a complete system or integrated into other styles of practice. The use of Ontake with MSA is an exciting new fusion of ideas that allows for even more creativity in clinical practice. Ontake can be applied at any of the four steps of treatment Dr Manaka defined.

Dr Manaka's octahedral model of the body, like everything else in his work, is not an abstract theoretical concept but a clinical model with intensely practical applications. His comprehensive and structured treatment approach applies the fundamental concepts of yin and yang to treatment. His four-step protocol which treats at both root and branch levels and has the additional aim of correcting structural abnormalities.

The first two steps comprise the root treatment. The remaining two steps address structural problems and branch treatment. Manaka described this approach as "looking for the most significant paradox in the body".[134]

Table 27. Manaka's Four Steps

Step 1	Identify and treat patterns of disharmony on the abdomen (yin surface).	Usually applied with polarity agents such as ion-pumping cords, electrostatic adsorbers, or Manaka's ion-beam device placed on the master and coupled points of the Eight Extras or the supplementing and draining points of the paired polar channels.
Step 2	Identify patterns of disharmony on the back (yang surface) related to the abdominal findings.	Most commonly applied with *kyutoshin* (warm needle) on the back-*shu* points related to the step 1 treatment, though simple *chishin* (retained needle) or even *okyu* (small cone moxibustion) can be substituted.
Step 3	Adjust structural imbalances through Sotai counter-resistance stretching exercises.	*Okyu* is often applied at the same time as the stretch.
Step 4	Control symptoms with moxibustion, additional retained needles, cupping, bloodletting, intradermal needling, tapping with Manaka's wooden needle and hammer, and/or Hirata Zone Therapy.	At this point, anything goes, provided it does not overtreat the patient. For an overview of Hirata Zone Therapy, see the end of this chapter.

134 Matsumoto, K., & Birch S. (1988). *Hara Diagnosis: Reflections on the Sea*, Brookline: Paradigm Publications.

We can think of this four-step protocol as a coat stand with four hooks. On each hook is a bag packed with one category of clothes: underwear, shirts, trousers and jackets. Every day, we rummage through each bag and take out one of each item, then we happily get dressed and go out. It doesn't matter which clothes we select, so long as they fulfil two criteria: they should fall into the broad categories above and they need to match each other.

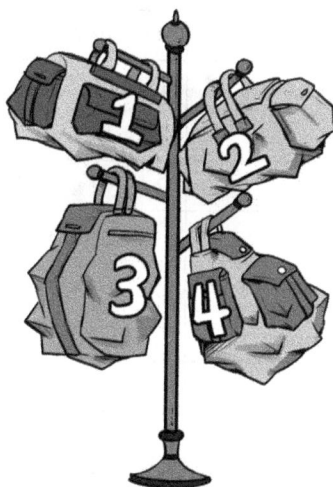

The four-step protocol provides us with four kitbags
of options, each with a clear objective.

Manaka's four-step system is the same. Our clinical kitbags contain a vast repertoire of techniques—needling, cupping, moxibustion, ear acupuncture, bloodletting, etc.—that may be used to treat our patients. Manaka simply reduced the process of treatment into four basic categories with stated objectives. You can hang any method you want on these four steps, as long as they meet the objectives. This chapter explores how we can integrate Ontake into steps 1–4.

Step 1—Releasing the Yin Aspect of the Body

The aim of Step 1 is to release pressure-pain findings on the abdomen, the anterior yin surface. Manaka's principal approach for this first step was his Eight Extraordinary Vessel treatment. The Eight Extras form an octahedral structure in the body, even from its embryological beginnings. Treatment is designed to restore equilibrium between these sections or quadrants, thus creating balance in the overall channel system. Manaka developed five basic patterns, which have been supplemented by patterns from instructors, such as Stephen Birch in Europe and Brenda Loew in the US, resulting in eight to ten commonly used patterns.

Table 27. Basic Patterns

Pattern	Master and couple points
Yin Qiao/Ren Mai	LU 7, KID 6
Chong Mai/Yin Wei Mai	P 6, SP 4
Yang Wei/Dai Mai	TB 5, GB 41
Yang Qiao/Du Mai	SI 3, BL 62
Cross Syndrome	P 6, SP 4 + TB 5, GB 41
Mixed Yin	LU 7, KID 6 + P 6, SP 4
K3L	LU 7, KID 6 + LI 4, LIV 3
Ren/Dai (Brenda pattern)	LU 7, KID 6 + TB 5, GB 41
Four Gates	LI 4, LIV 3

In addition to these basic patterns, there are quite a few other patterns based on abdominal reactions that can be applied. Manaka also used polar channel pairs, treating the supplementing and draining points of both channels with polarity agents.

Table 28 Polar channel pair treatment points

	Supplementing	Draining		Supplementing	Draining
Lung	LU 9+	LU 5–	**Bladder**	BL 67+	BL 65–
Large intestine	LI 11+	LI 2–	**Kidney**	KID 7+	KID 1–
Stomach	ST 41+	ST 45–	**Pericardium**	P 9+	P 7–
Spleen	SP2+	SP5–	**Triple burner**	TB 3+	TB 10–
Heart	HT 9+	HT 7–	**Gall bladder**	GB 43+	GB 38–
Small intestine	SI 3+	SI 8–	**Liver**	LIV 8+	LIV 2–

Ontake During Step 1

Ontake can be applied for the following purposes:
- Releasing stubborn reactions on the abdomen when the cords are in place
- Treating symptoms when the cords are in place
- As a non-pattern-based root treatment when ion pumping at Step 1 is not appropriate

Ontake for Stubborn Reactions

Sometimes when using ion-pumping cords, there is a general improvement on the abdomen, but some stubborn reactions remain unchanged. Manaka described three such situations and designated points to use for each one.

Ontake can be used as another method of releasing these stubborn reactions. The principle is to tap along the channel of the master and couple points, at the appropriate frequency. As we saw in chapter 8, using the channels of the master and coupled points also affects the octahedron, resulting in a different "flavour" of the Eight Extras.

Table 29. Manaka's Points for Stubborn Reactions and Ontake Variations

Stubborn Reaction Point	Manaka's Recommended Distal Point	Ontake Distal Treatment
KID 16	KID 7 (ipsilateral)	Tap from KID 3 to KID 10 (120)
Subcostal	LIV 8 (ipsilateral)	Roll at LIV 8 (108) or Taking care to avoid the needle at P 6, tap P 3 to P 7 (176) and SP 5 to SP 9 (132).
ASIS	SP 6 (ipsilateral)	Tap SP 5 to SP 9 (132).

All three points suggested by Manaka are on the leg. This is because points higher up on the body can induce counterflow qi reactions when the ion-pumping cords are connected, not because of the actions of the points themselves, but because of the introduction of a metal needle to the circuit. Ontake, being made of wood, does not have the same effect, and I have used it on upper body points on the body routinely while the cords are in place.

This principle of treating the related channels can be used to target any stubborn reaction, not just the three described by Manaka. Thus, any of the basic patterns, or any of the polar channel pairs can be treated in this way. For example, if treating a large intestine/kidney pattern, then tap along the large intestine and kidney channels (108 and 120). When needling the points on the polar channel pairs, it is advisable to tape the needles in place with micropore so the vibration of the Ontake doesn't dislodge them.

This simple method has proved so effective at releasing stubborn reactions that it became the inspiration for the BB-8 whole body treatment described in chapter 8.

Inspired by Japanese author and trainer Kiiko Matsumoto, who observed "gummy" areas on the arm and leg that release the belly when needled, here are two additional strategies that are effective with Ontake for clearing stubborn abdominal reactions.

Table 30. Matsumoto Reactions and Ontake Variations

Stubborn Reaction Points	Matsumoto's Recommended Distal Points	Ontake Distal Treatment
Left ST 25 to ST-27 (*oketsu* area)	Left LIV 4, left LU 5	Roll above and below these two points at 108 and 126 bpm, respectively.
Right ST 25 to ST-27 (immune area)	"Triple Intestine" 10	Palpate for reactions at the level of LI 10 and roll (108), extending to the median aspect onto the triple burner channel (152).

Treating the Branch

If using ion-pumping cords and needles, treatment usually takes about ten minutes. This provides a ten-minute window during which we can apply other supplementary treatments, either at the root level, as above, or at the branch level. Manaka's four steps do not need to be applied sequentially; they can be applied concurrently. It is, therefore, entirely acceptable to apply Ontake branch treatments or pain-relieving treatments during Step 1. For example, if treating a patient with urinary issues presenting with a YQR pattern, we can easily use the time to apply Ontake on the lower Ren points to supplement the lower burner.

If treating a patient with lower back pain on the left, (posterior lower left quadrant) presenting with a cross syndrome, we can apply Ontake to the anterior right upper quadrant (see chapter 11). If a patient has diarrhoea or constipation, we can apply Ontake around the navel (see chapter 9).

Non-Pattern-Based Root Treatments (NPBRT)

Sometimes Manaka would choose not to use his ion-pumping cord treatments at Step 1 and instead apply a whole-body moxa treatment. In some situations, particularly when faced with a challenging diagnosis, it may be useful to apply a whole-body root treatment with Ontake such as Bamboo Max or BB-8, both described in chapter 8.

Step 1 is the patient's first contact with your treatment methods: they may often be a little stressed or anxious at this point, perhaps because it is their first treatment or because they were rushing to be on time for the appointment. Sitting in the waiting area, they still feel connected to their work or family issues through their mobile devices. They may be in physical or emotional pain. Thus, Step 1 should be the time to bring them from this initial state of tension to a more relaxed state so they can receive the information from the treatment.

When teaching, Stephen Birch has said that he sometimes favours ion-pumping cords with needles over some of the faster polarity devices such as electrostatic adsorbers. This is because the longer process required by needling "pins down" the patient for ten minutes, and that stillness encourages them to relax. We can, therefore, add to Manaka's goal Step 1:

Release the yin aspect of the body and help the patient to relax.

Ontake can help do this very quickly.

Step 2—Releasing the Yang Aspect of the Body

If the aim of Step 1 is to release the yin aspect of the body and help the patient relax, the aim of Step 2 is to release the yang aspect of the body, principally the back. In classical MSA, Step 2 involves locating reactions at the back-*shu* points that relate to the abdominal diagnosis. For example, when treating the Yang Wei–Dai Mai pair with ion-pumping cords on the master and coupled points TB 5 and GB 41, the corresponding step 2 treatment would be BL 19 and BL 22, the back-*shu* points of the gall bladder and triple burner. Usually, Manaka used *kyutoshin* (warm needle) technique, or if the patient was thin and unsuitable for the deeper needling required, he would use *chishin* (shallow needling) and a heat lamp.

Ontake can be of great use here. First of all, adapting the Bamboo Mini treatment to Step 2 is simple. Rather than looking for reactions specifically at the back-*shu* points relating to the Step 1 treatment, Bamboo Mini addresses all the reactions along the bladder line from BL 11 to BL 30, as well as along the Du Mai. Thus, Ontake can be used in a very simple way to treat all the back-*shu* points and achieve the goal of Step 2.

Manaka's Reactive Points

Manaka also suggested that another way to release the yang aspect of the body is to examine and treat reactions on the yang channels. Since examining every yang point for reactions is time-consuming, Manaka provided a list of points that he commonly found to be reactive. Needling just one to three of these points can be very effective in Step 2.[135]

Table 31 Manaka's reactive points

Large Intestine	4, 10, 11, 15, 16, 18, 19, 20
Stomach	3, 6, 7, 8, 9, 11, 12
Small intestine	3, 7, 9, 11, 14, 18, 19
Bladder	2, 7, 9, 10, 11, 12
Triple burner	5, 8, 13, 14, 17, 20, 21
Gall bladder	2, 7, 12, 14, 20, 21
Governor vessel	10, 12, 14, 15, 20, 23

We have seen that Ontake can be used to treat an entire channel very quickly. In the Bamboo Max treatment, treating all three arm yang channels is a quick procedure. When treating the arm, attention can be focused on Manaka's list of points above. On the leg, the bladder and gall bladder channels can be treated as part of the Bamboo Mini treatment. Simple tapping along the bladder and gall bladder channels at their respective frequencies releases the yang aspect of the body, achieving the goal of Step 2.

Channel Stretches with Moxa

Manaka described another treatment method called channel stretches (also known as stretch moxa) that is applicable either at Step 2, to release the yang channels, or at Step 4, for symptom relief. This is discussed at length in *Chasing the Dragon's Tail*:

A third treatment style that is applicable to step two treatments is the use of either the fire needle or moxa on reactive channel points while the patient

---

135   Manaka, Y., Itaya, K., & Birch, S. (1995). *Chasing the Dragon's Tail: The Theory and Practice of Acupuncture in the Work of Yoshio Manaka*. Brookline: Paradigm Publications, p. 188.

stretches the appropriate channel and exhales. This is effective for releasing tension or stagnation in the lung, large intestine, triple burner, and small intestine channels, four channels that are typically involved in neck-shoulder stiffness problems…

It is good both for the symptomatic relief of neck and shoulder problems; and for the release of functional tensions and obstructions in these regions. By itself, it may be the complete second step of treatment, or it may be used together with *kyutoshin* on the back associated-shu points. It can be applicable later in step four treatment for the relief of symptoms on the shoulder, neck, and other dorsal areas.[136]

Clearly, Manaka was not doctrinaire about *kyutoshin* (warm needle) during Step 2. For him, the objective was always most important, not the method used to achieve it. Any appropriate tool in the kitbag would do. Thus, channel stretching could be used as a complete Step 2 treatment, and of course, Ontake is a good substitute for fire needle or moxa.

The key difference between using Ontake in this context and the fire needle or small cone moxibustion used by Manaka is the way the patient perceives the heat. When applying cone moxa, she feels nothing for the first few seconds, and then there is a little "pinch" of heat when we extinguish the moxa. The same is true for the fire needle: she feels nothing until the hot tip momentarily touches her skin. These two techniques cause a moment of discomfort, which induces a contraction or fasciculation in the muscle, allowing it to relax and lengthen.

To create a similar moment of discomfort with Ontake, we need to reverse our prior thinking about it. Typically, with a technique like Standing, we make sure we don't leave the Ontake in one place long enough for the patient to feel discomfort. For stretch moxa (and for Sotai in Step 3), we now need to perform the opposite. We want the bamboo to be freshly lit, so the plug is glowing red hot, and we want to stand it on the point until the patient reports that it feels too hot.

Don't worry! Even with a freshly lit and glowing Ontake, the initial sensation is comfortable warmth unless you have heated the lip and skin of the bamboo by mistake. Within a few seconds, however, as we hold the lighted end in place, the heat builds up until it feels too much. It is at this moment of discomfort that we simultaneously release the stretch and remove the bamboo.

With this Ontake variation, however, the interaction with the patient is reversed from normal channel stretching. In normal channel stretching, we tell the patient

---

136 Ibid., p. 191.

to drop the stretch and relax as we extinguish the moxa. In this case, we instruct the patient to say "Now!", as soon as the bamboo feels too hot. At the same time, she should release the stretch. As she does this, we simultaneously remove the bamboo. So, in normal classical stretching, we control the heat and the moment of release. In Ontake channel stretching, the patient controls the heat and the moment of release.

Channel Stretching on the Small Intestine

In *Chasing the Dragon's Tail*, Manaka describes channel stretches to the lung, large intestine, triple burner, and small intestine channels.[137] As an illustrative example, below is a description of stretching the small intestine channel using Ontake.[138] These exercises can bring about dramatic and immediate changes to the shoulders and neck, significantly increasing range of motion.

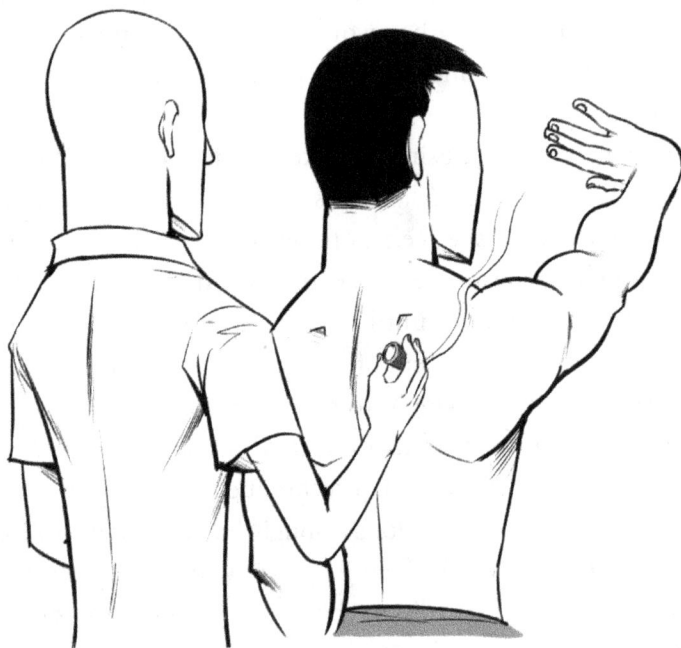

Channel stretching with Ontake (small intestine).

You need to explain the procedure to your patients before you start the exercise. It is always good to do a dummy run, without heat, until they feel confident they know what you intend them to do.

---

137 Ibid., pp. 191–193.

138 Adapted from Channel Stretch handout written together with my colleague and co-trainer Marian Fixler.

1. Ask your patient to extend her arm forwards with her wrist rotated medially and dorsiflexed to ninety degrees, or as close as possible. Check the following points for tenderness: SI 9, SI 10, and SI 11.

2. Once you have identified the most tender point, rest your hand near the point, holding the Ontake away from it.

3. Ask the patient to inhale as she stretches the channel as described above. Ask her to hold her breath, and at the same time, place the lighted mouth of the Ontake on the point.

4. As soon as she feels the heat is uncomfortable, usually three to five seconds, she should breathe out loudly or say "Now!" while dropping her arm. At the same time, you should quickly remove the Ontake.

5. Repeat this procedure three times, re-palpating for tenderness each time.

Variation

Manaka developed a variation of channel stretching using his wooden needle and hammer. You can emulate this with Ontake by putting the bamboo on its side and knocking hard with a knuckle. The warmth of the bamboo increases the percussive effect of the knocking.

When on its side, the bamboo may not feel so hot, so usually you can keep knocking for a maximum of eight beats. If the bamboo skin is very thin, as is the case if it's been used a long time, it may get hot enough to cause discomfort, so you should still ask her to say "Now!" if it gets too hot. Thus, for Step 4 below, you need to be flexible and prepared for two options, listed below as option (a.) or (b.).

1. Ask her to extend her arm forwards with her wrist rotated medially and dorsiflexed to ninety degrees, or as close as possible. Check the following points for tenderness: SI 9, SI 10, and SI 11.

2. Once you have identified the most tender point, place the Ontake on its side on the point and ask the patient to stretch her arm more and inhale.

3. Ask her to hold her breath as she continues the stretch. At the same time, start knocking on the Ontake at the point's frequency.

4. Follow the method which arises naturally:
    a. When she calls out "Now!", exhaling and relaxing her arm, remove the Ontake immediately.
    b. Continue knocking for a maximum of eight beats, finishing with an extra hard knock on the last beat. At the same time, ask her to exhale, and drop her arm.

5. Repeat this procedure three times, re-palpating for tenderness each time.

Playing Chicken

Recently I was treating a patient with severe neck pain using channel stretching on the small intestine and triple burner channels. I used the first of the above methods with Ontake. Interestingly, he was sensitive to heat on the healthy side but quite insensitive to heat on the problem side. For this reason, the session became a game of chicken!

As he was not giving me any indication that he could feel the heat, at some point I felt I had held the hot bamboo on his skin for quite long enough, and I intervened, removing the bamboo and asking him to breathe out and drop his arm.

This is a common-sense point to make, but it's worth highlighting. At no stage should you hold the burning bamboo on the patient's skin long enough to cause a burn. Whether the patient is insensitive or trying to be brave, if there is a game of chicken afoot, the practitioner should always blink first.

His reaction to the treatment is worth sharing. Even though he has severe prolapse in several cervical vertebrae, he felt great pain relief and left the session on a high.

Step 3—Treating Structural Imbalances

Manaka described Step 3 as optional, and he routinely did not include it in the treatment flow for patients, reserving it only for when the patient showed clear structural imbalances. Such imbalances may be differences in tightness at the hips when comparing left and right, or the muscles on one side of the spine might be more developed than the other.

Sotai

Manaka studied, incorporated, and modified a series of exercises known as Sotai. Sotai was first developed by Keizo Hashimoto (1897–1993) and involves using counter-resistance stretches to release restrictions of movement.[139] Manaka found ways to improve and adapt the therapy by incorporating the application of heat during the counter-resistance stretches. Sometimes using fire needling, but usually small cone moxibustion, he noted that the sudden pinch of heat from these tools greatly enhanced the effect of the exercises.

---

139 Hashimoto, K., & Kawakami, Y. (1983). *Sotai: Balance and Health Through Natural Movement*. Tokyo: Japan Publications Inc.

Manaka's Sotai routines with moxa are discussed in detail in *Chasing the Dragon's Tail*.[140] Manaka also described how two practitioners could apply Sotai together, one performing the stretch and resistance, the other tapping on the treatment point with a wooden hammer and needle at the appropriate frequency.

In another variation, the practitioner rocks the wooden needle in time to the metronome with one hand while performing the stretch with the other. With Manaka's precedents already in place to apply Step 3 with heat, pressure, percussion, or rocking at the appropriate meridian frequency, it is easy to extrapolate new variations with Ontake.

As with channel stretching above, the principal difference between Ontake, fire needle, or cone moxa is timing the perception of heat. When applying cone moxa, nothing is felt for the first few seconds, and then there is a little "pinch" of heat as we extinguish it, simultaneously giving the command to stop pushing. With Ontake, when we hold the bamboo to the skin, a comfortable warmth is felt immediately, but as we hold the lighted end in place, the heat builds up over a few seconds until it feels too much. This is the moment to simultaneously to release the resistance and remove the bamboo. Thus, the procedure is the reverse of normal Sotai with moxa. Instead of telling the patient to relax as we extinguish the moxa, we should instruct the patient to call out "Now!" when she feels the heat is uncomfortable, and that is the moment when we remove the bamboo and release our resistance to the limb and let it relax.

Procedure

The most commonly used Sotai stretch in MSA is Prone Leg Flexion, which is usually taught on the first weekend of a Manaka course. Using this particular technique as an example, here is a way to integrate Ontake.[141] As a general rule, it is always better with Sotai to explain the procedure and do one or two dummy runs without heat before starting the exercise for real.

---

140 Manaka, Y., Itaya, K., & Birch, S. (1995). *Chasing the Dragon's Tail: The Theory and Practice of Acupuncture in the Work of Yoshio Manaka*. Brookline: Paradigm Publications, pp. 196–203.

141 Adapted from a Sotai handout written together with my colleague and co-trainer, Marian Fixler.

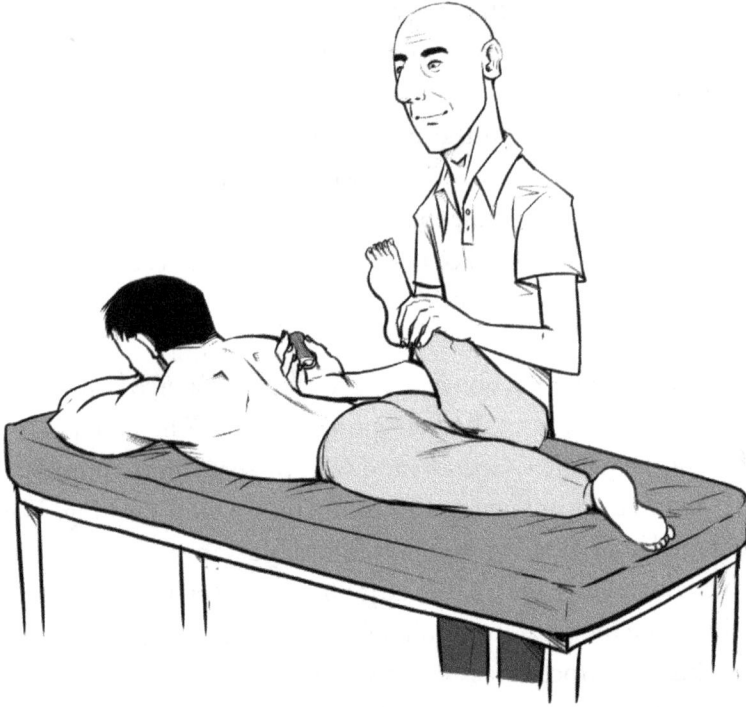

1. Hold the bamboo near BL 18 and bring the leg just past the point of resistance.

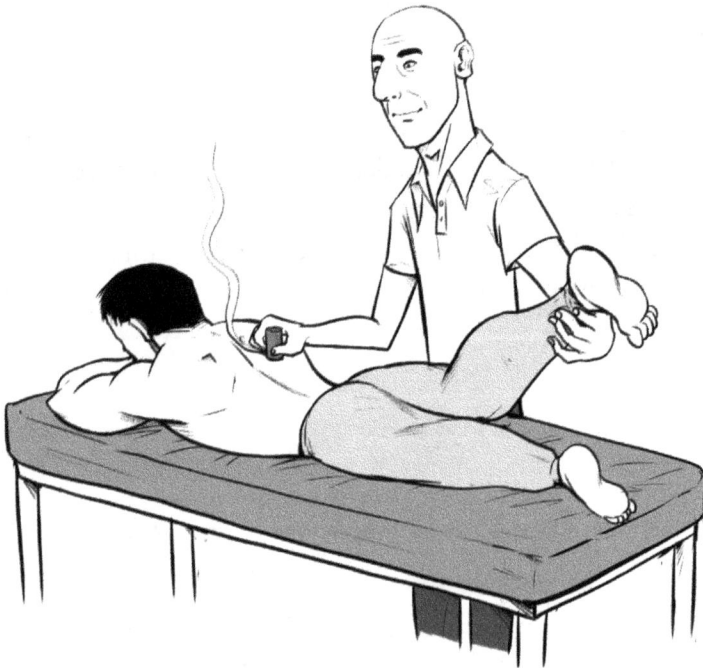

2. Rest the lighted end of the Ontake on the point and ask the patient to push against resistance. Remove and release on the patient's command.

1. *Doshin:* Examine the patient for restricted movement and asymmetries in muscle tone. With the patient lying prone, stretch both legs towards the buttocks.

2. Assess which side is less restricted. Perform the exercise initially on the more flexible side. It is common to do the exercise twice on the healthier side and once on the more restricted side.

3. Palpate for a tight point around BL 18. Place the bamboo near the point, holding it as you would for tapping, but keep the lighted end away from the skin. Ask the patient to inhale, move her leg to the point of resistance, then stretch it just a little bit more towards the buttocks, without causing discomfort. Now extend the leg slowly, asking the patient to exhale as you move it away from the restriction.

4. Just before her leg is fully extended, get the patient to push gently against your hand while applying resistance to the movement. At the same time, rest the lighted end of the bamboo against BL 18 and instruct the patient to say "Now!" when the heat is no longer comfortable.

5. When the patient says "Now!", remove the bamboo, relax the counter-resistance, and let the patient completely relax her leg.

6. Reassess the movement to determine the efficacy of your treatment.

Note: This procedure is not performed in time to a metronome.

Variation

Manaka's mastered a one-handed application with the wooden needle. In this variation, Manaka rocked the wooden needle on the point in time to the metronome. In the same way, Ontake can be rolled, rocked, pressed, or vibrated on the point at the appropriate frequency while the stretch is applied with the other hand. With this variation, there is no intention to create a moment of discomfort with the bamboo. Instead, we are relying on the warmth and the frequency to relax the point.

Hirata Zone Therapy

Before discussing Step 4, it is time for a final brief discussion of a system that Manaka used very often: Hirata Zone Therapy (HZT).

The Hirata zone system of correspondences is a Japanese holographic system of treatment about which little has been written in English. It is based on the work of Kurakichi Hirata (1901–1945), who studied medicine at Kyoto Teikoku University in the 1930s and developed his own system of heated needle treatment while there.

Dr Manaka was an exponent of HZT and forty years after Hirata's death wrote his own book on the subject. He used the method frequently, particularly at Step 4 as an adjunctive treatment.

Hirata saw the skin as the place where humans interface with the natural world. This is the place where diseases enter and where reactions take place. For this reason, he emphasised diagnosing and treating at the skin level, and he developed a method for stimulating the skin with a heated tool.

Hirata's theory was quite simple. He developed a medicalised hologram composed of twelve horizontal zones (see below). These twelve zones are mapped out in six different regions, the head, face, neck, torso, arms and legs. Zones in each region are isophasal with the same zone in another region. For example, someone with kidney disease may have reactions in the kidney zones beneath the eye, at the wrist, and in the knees. By stimulating each kidney zone, where the kidney organ manifests on the skin, he thought he could improve the condition and function of the kidney itself.

Although there are twelve zones that largely correspond to the twelve channels, there are no correspondences for the triple burner or pericardium. Instead, there are new correspondences for the bronchi and the reproductive organs. The gall bladder zone and spleen zone also reflect and treat the exocrine and endocrine functions of the pancreas, respectively:

1. Bronchi
2. Lungs
3. Heart
4. Liver
5. Gall bladder and exocrine gland of the pancreas
6. Spleen and endocrine gland of the pancreas
7. Stomach
8. Kidney
9. Large intestine
10. Small intestine
11. Bladder
12. Reproductive organs

Hirata's rationale for the zones was that each region is a hologram of the body. Therefore, each region will reflect the same physiological and pathological processes in the same way. An imbalance in the liver organ, for example, will manifest in reactions on the liver zone in each region.

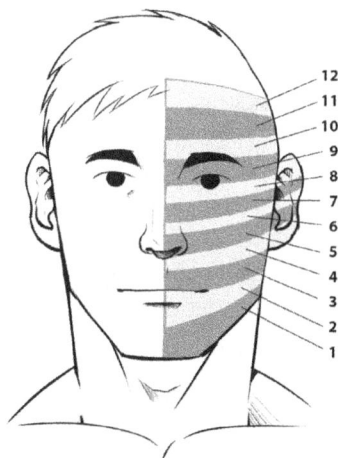

The twelve Hirata zones on the face region.

Therapeutic Uses

HZT involves stimulating zones with a heated blunt probe. In the old days, this was a cone-shaped metal instrument, lined with asbestos and filled with burning ethyl alcohol, called the *shinryoki*, or "Mind Therapy Device". In keeping with his mission to empower self-treatment, this device was distributed for free with his first bestselling book. Many years later, Dr Manaka developed an electrically heated roller called the *tenshin kyu*. Contemporary Hirata practitioners use a more sophisticated electronic hot probe called the *Hirata-kun*.[142] These heated tools are used to tap or roll on the appropriate Hirata zones until they turn red.

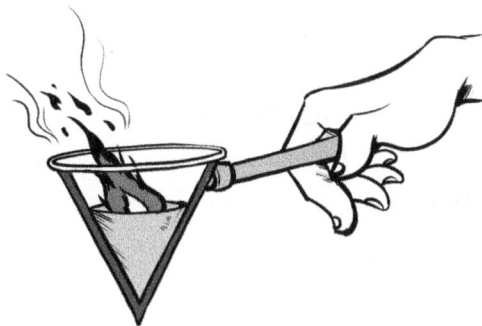

Hirata's original heated needle or *shinryoki*.

---

142 *Hirata-shiki Nesshin Ryoho Setsumeisho (Hirata-style Warm Needle Therapy Instruction Booklet.* Tokyo: Kokusai Nihon Onnetsu Ryoho Kenkyukai (International Japanese Thermotherapy) Association), p. 9.

These devices are either no longer available or, in the case of the *Hirata-kun*, prohibitively expensive. Over the last two years, however, I have used Ontake as a substitute heat source with great success. This work led to the integration of Hirata Zone Therapy into my Manaka practice and a long, detailed written examination of how to apply it with Ontake, which will appear in a second book devoted solely to Hirata and Ontake.

This is an exciting project, so exciting it is impossible to resist teasing it here! It breathes new life into the teachings of both Hirata and Manaka and considerably broadens the scope of Ontake from what has been possible before.

In terms of integration, HZT can be applied with Ontake as an adjunctive treatment at any of Manaka's four steps. Stephen Birch provides some instruction on the zones in *Chasing the Dragon's Tail* and *Hara Diagnosis—Reflections on the Sea*.

Step 4—Anything Goes

Although this book has explored Ontake's use in the realm of Step 1, it is in Step 4 that it really comes into its own. As we have seen in the preceding chapters, Ontake can be applied to treat the branch in a variety of ways, adapting very simplistic approaches such as "put it where it hurts because it feels good", adaptations of established moxibustion protocols such as Fukaya's, and very sophisticated distal holographic models such as those developed by Tan and Hirata.

You can apply Ontake for Step 4 during Step 1 or Step 2, or it can be the last thing you do before the end of the session. Ontake is such a versatile tool that in the realm of Step 4, anything goes.

Summary

Ontake can be used at every stage of Manaka's four-step treatment process, treating stubborn reactions at Steps 1 and 2 and helping with structural adjustment Step 3. At Step 4, everything we have explored in all the previous chapters can be adapted. By doing so, we add new layers to MSA, often substituting Ontake for needling and making the whole experience feel lighter and subtler.

I hope that readers understand from the above that it can be an equally simple matter to integrate Ontake into your system of acupuncture, whatever that style may be.

The next and final chapter of this book looks to the future, both for readers of this book and for Ontake.

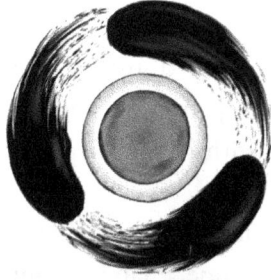

CHAPTER 14

FOLLOWING MANAKA'S TRAIL

Providing simple advice for practitioners and a
"who's who" of the contemporary world of Ontake.

The Ontake Method

This book has introduced one of the newest tools in acupuncture. Bamboo has been around for perhaps fifty years. The Ontake Method, the integrated techniques described in this book, has been around for fewer than ten.

Ontake treats only at the level of the skin, what Hirata saw as the all-important interface between the environment and our inner world. In the trigram of Heaven, Person, and Earth, the influence of heaven and earth enters our body through the skin. Here lies the power of Ontake. Rather than treating acupuncture points, it mostly treats regions, zones, and lines.

Despite this broad regional application, Ontake can easily target specific symptoms, channels, or organ systems, and it has a broad range of effects that treat the body holistically. While it historically has been used as a branch tool, it can be used to treat the root or as a supplement to root treatment.

Ontake is different from most moxibustion tools in that it can be used percussively, as a rolling tool, or for deep friction and pressing. This makes it extremely versatile, allowing it to be used with Manaka's meridian frequencies to act at different levels.

The integration of holographic systems, such as those used by Dr Tan, Dr Manaka and Hirata, adds new range and scope, enabling Ontake to treat pain and functional disorders as part of the branch component of treatment.

By bringing together such a wide variety of practices and concepts, Ontake is a wonderful combination of ancient and modern. Moxibustion itself is ancient, but Ontake is a new way to apply it. Ontake is like a new branch, and with the completion of this book, it should be fully grafted onto the Western tree of contemporary acupuncture. Like a proud gardener, I am enjoying watching its new shoots grow and spread. Bamboo has been such a friend to Asian civilisation, used in hundreds of different ways. Here we have found yet another.

Many fresh ideas and applications for Ontake are bound to develop in the future. To paraphrase Winston Churchill, this is not the end of the Ontake story. It is not even the beginning of the end. But it is, perhaps, the end of the beginning. For such a simple device—just a tiny piece of bamboo filled with moxa wool—it is abundant with possibilities.

Other Approaches to Ontake

Ten years ago, there were only a handful of practitioners in Japan using what was then called short bamboo. As a result of articles by various practitioners and the instant transmission of social media, its popularity has grown in this short time, not just in Japan, but also in the West. I personally have taught Ontake in the UK, Spain, Croatia, Japan, Malaysia, Indonesia, Thailand, Israel, and Brazil and have corresponded with Ontake practitioners in the US, Australia, New Zealand, France, Germany, and Chile.

In Japan, Yamashita's legacy is taking root, with teachers who studied with him disseminating his ideas in classes and on YouTube. Bamboo Tube Moxibustion is now covered, albeit briefly, at Toyo Shinkyu Senmon Gakkoh, one of the foremost acupuncture schools in Tokyo. Clearly, many people are adopting this tool worldwide.

Here is a summary of other practitioners practising Ontake in their own ways. I am sure there are others doing exciting things whom I have not yet encountered.

Susumu Honda

Tokyo-based practitioner Susumu Honda has refined the original design of Ontake by winding a strip of lead around the top end to increase its weight. He calls this model the Ontake Pro. The lead ring brings the total weight of the Ontake Pro to about one hundred100 grams. The extra weight of the lead gives it a solidity that makes tapping very even and penetrating. Honda gives the Ontake Pro to patients for home use. "This frees the handler "from worry about the tapping strength and recreates the soothing, rhythmical *kata tataki* tapping." [143]

The Ontake Pro can be used for the applications described in this book, particularly those that require more percussive strokes. However, with a ring of lead at one end, its shape is asymmetrical, so it cannot easily be used on its side for rolling. Honda gives the Ontake Pro to patients for home use.

Hideo Shinma

The son of the renowned moxibustion practitioner Isaburo Fukaya (1901–1974), Hideo Shinma is an accomplished classical guitar player in his eighties. He is also working hard to preserve and pass on his father's legacy by writing and teaching in collaboration with acupuncturist and teacher Tetsuya Fukushima. With his booklet *Take Zutsu Onkyu*, Shinma became one of the first to write about "Bamboo Tube Moxibustion.[144]

His approach is to use Ontake as a local treatment for the branch—for example, treating the sacrum and buttocks area for sciatica. He has adapted many of Fukaya's moxa principles, looking for abnormal tissue findings such as indurations and treating them with Ontake instead of *tonnetsukyu* (hot moxibustion).

A dedicated pipe smoker, his book also describes substituting his favourite pipe for Ontake (it is unclear if it's filled with moxa or tobacco!) and rubbing with that instead. Smoking pipes actually make perfect heat application tools, particularly for rubbing the skin, as the sides of the pipe are highly polished.

Felip Caudet

Felip Caudet is a physiotherapist and practitioner of moxibustion based in Catalonia, Spain. An ardent exponent of Fukaya-style moxibustion and one who frequently visits Japan to study with Fukushima Sensei and Shinma Sensei, he has developed

---

143 Honda, S. (2017). Ontake and Iron Stick Moxibustion. *NAJOM*, 24 (69).
144 Shinma, H. (2012). *Take Zutsu Onkyu*. Tokyo: Kyuho Rinsho Kenkyukai.

kinseikyu, a method of postural assessment and adjustment using moxibustion on indurations along the fascial chains.

After a postural assessment, *kinseikyu* involves three steps of treatment: first; *okyu* (small cone moxibustion), then treatment along the muscle chain with Ontake, and finally fascial stretching. In *kinseikyu*, the bamboo tube typically is longer, aptly named Superontake (see chapter 2).

The bamboo is applied with variations on the techniques described in this book, such as tapping, rolling, or vibrating. In this context, Ontake is used as a supplementary treatment following small cone moxibustion.

Hideto Onuki

Hideto Onuki is a practitioner of acupuncture and moxibustion based in Tokyo. He was introduced to *takenowa kyu* (Bamboo Ring Moxibustion) in a short class at his college, Toyo Shinkyu Senmon Gakkoh in Tokyo, and was taught to use it as a simple heat application tool, applying it locally. As *deshi* to Masao Togasaki, a well-known teacher of *Yawarakai Shiki Chiryo* (Royal Touch Style), he learnt to use skin palpation to classify acupuncture points into four kinds of reaction.

Onuki has integrated bamboo into this style, using it in very subtle ways to balance *kyo* and *jitsu* findings at different levels of the skin and soft tissue. He currently uses it primarily for its local effects rather than systemically. When treating indurations, he uses it to warm and soften, varying the pressure according to depth and feel. When the skin is loose and flabby, he applies it slowly, gradually inserting the heat. For inflammation and pain, he uses a kind of rubbing technique to disperse the pain. He uses moxibustion, needles, or Ontake interchangeably, depending on the situation. He considers it particularly suitable to use it with children and sensitive patients.

Mika Takano

Mika Takano is a moxibustion practitioner with a unique approach. She specialises in women's health and working with couples trying to conceive. Based in Chiba, near Tokyo, she works predominantly with Ontake and platform moxa. She aims to regulate the surface of the body and is influenced by concepts of regulation, such as Junji Mizutani's "ground levelling", discussed in chapter 3.[145]

---

145   Mizutani, J. (2018, May 30). Interview by Oran Kivity with Stephen Birch, Junji Mizutani, and Brenda Loew. Retrieved from https://youtu.be/aoN3bwXmacY

Although trained in acupuncture, she chooses not to use pulse taking, *hara* diagnosis, conventional meridian theory, or textbook acupuncture points. This means that her therapy relies principally on very sensitive skin palpation and identifying and treating abnormal tissue findings in areas and points. She uses Ontake to regulate— essentially balancing *kyo* and *jitsu* on the surface—and then applies platform moxa on the abdomen. Ontake treatment comes first, both as a way to put patients at ease and to soften the overall musculature. Treatment is in two stages, first supine, then prone, with an emphasis on palpation to identify the areas and points for treatment. Sometimes these points end up corresponding to standard acupuncture points or points suggested by Fukaya. Ontake treatment usually finishes on the sole of the feet, to stop energy rising to the head.

Takano makes her own Ontake, smaller than the standard size, and when loading with moxa, she uses a shorter plug that creates less heat, similar to Shinma's methods. By working purely with moxa, she is creating a "moxa salon" or "*okyu* shop", and she feels she is reproducing the ancient model of moxibustion as a home therapy and people's medicine.

How Do I Integrate Ontake into My Practice?

The answer to this question is not complicated. With any skill, learning comes from doing. Reading a book is one thing, but Ontake and its applications with meridian frequency moxibustion are so intensely practical that the true lessons come from doing it. This book has examined uses for Ontake at root, branch, and supplementary levels. Depending on your own experience and understanding, some of these uses may resonate more with you than others. Those are the places to start. Start with what you have easily grasped, and when you feel ready, move on to those uses that initially seemed more challenging. Practise with colleagues and friends. If you have questions, join the Facebook group on Ontake and feel free to ask questions.

If it was not completely obvious by now, I love Ontake! It has transformed my practice. Most importantly, patients love it, and this was a huge part of its successful integration—apart from its effectiveness as a clinical tool. It is also small, light, cheap, and easy to apply. Whatever theories you use or styles of acupuncture you practice, it can easily be brought into play without a major shift in your way of working.

Shu-Ha-Ri—Following Manaka's Trail

In Chasing the Dragon's Tail, we are presented with the calligraphic image of Shu-Ha-Ri, which described the Buddhist concept of "the path" (michi) reflected in the many aspects of Japanese culture. In great brevity here, shu or mamoru means to protect, preserve and copy faithfully the teaching one receives. Ha means to detach, or in practical terms, to practice the art and technique in your own life, where you discover the limits and particular uses of the techniques you so faithfully learned. Ri means to leave, or separate—where one allows their own experience, intuition and personality to truly direct their own path.

Dr. Manaka followed the teachings of Shu-Ha-Ri, as perhaps all mavericks do. ... In the end, we can say that Dr. Manaka belongs, not to Japan, but to the world, and the complete study of his role in the evolution of a truly integrated medicine remains to be documented.

—Jeffrey Dann[146]

Chasing the Dragon's Tail, Manaka's landmark work in English, was published in 1989 shortly after his death. Since then, Stephen Birch has written shorter pieces about Manaka in other books and publications, but essentially no new books about Manaka's methods of treatment have been published in thirty years. Although he is still highly regarded as an influential acupuncturist, much of his written work has been forgotten—even in Japan—and contemporary students are not encouraged to study him or his methods.

I never had the privilege to meet this unique thinker and great man, but I feel that he influenced me in many significant ways, not least through passing on his "curiosity virus" to my teacher Stephen Birch. For many years, I have practised Manaka-style acupuncture in the ways that I was taught, but with Ontake, I found an opportunity to expand the limits of what I learnt. What's more, this wonderful tool has given me a chance to explore and breathe new life into the teachings of Hirata, which were never fully revealed to the West.

As a student of Dr Manaka's work, I would love to believe that he would have been delighted to find his ideas extended in these new directions. Most certainly, he would have delighted in playing with such a simple new heat device as Ontake. I have no doubt he would have come up with all kinds of modifications and adaptations that would push its range of uses far beyond the ones I have so far developed. As Ontake develops a life of its own, I hope that with this book, others will develop Manaka's ideas in different directions, grasping and following Manaka's trail.

---

146 Dann, J. (2009). Editorial. *NAJOM, 16*(47).

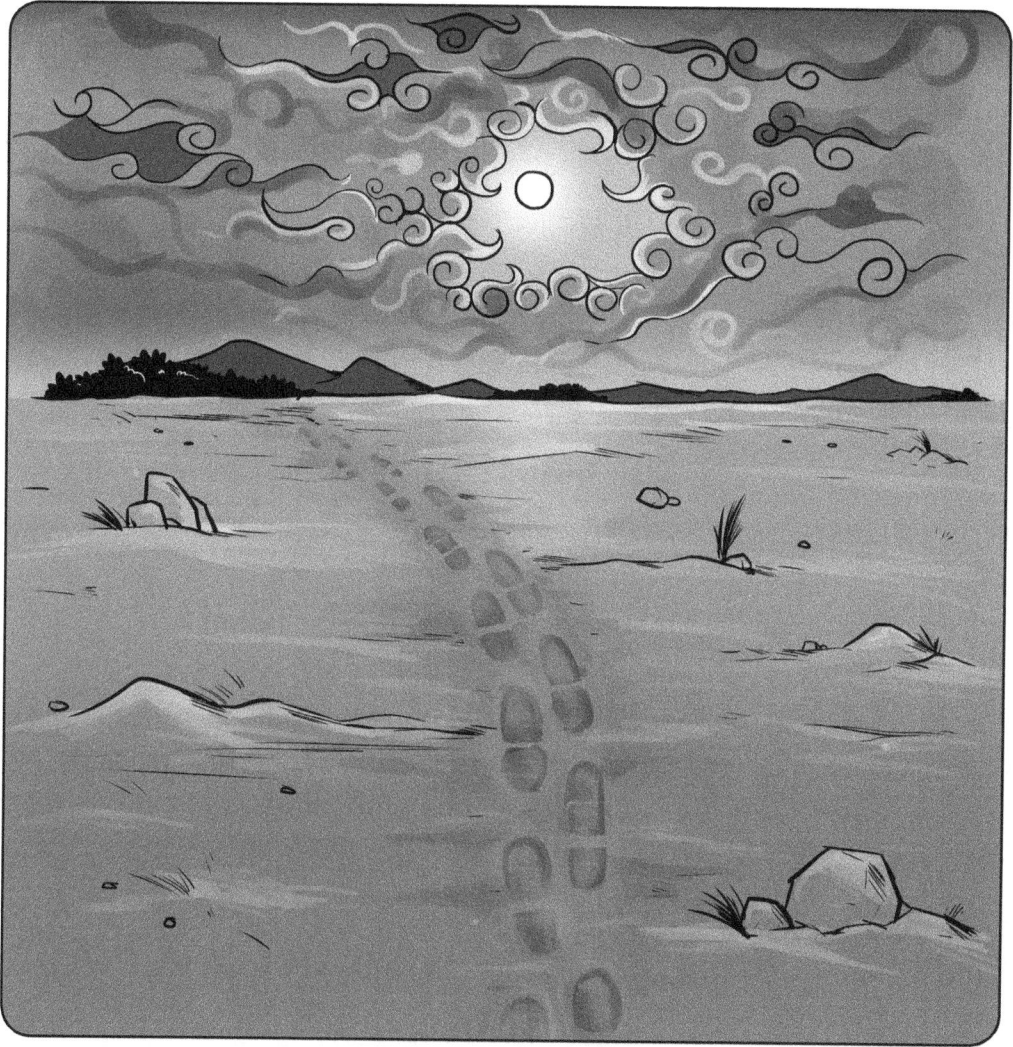

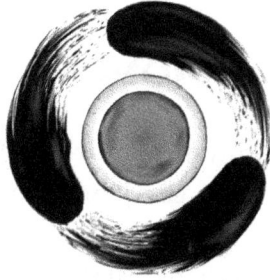

APPENDIX RESOURCE LIST

SUPPLIES

Ontake Myojo moxa wool	Both normal and Superontake are available at Sankei acupuncture suppliers, Tokyo. The owner, Hiroshi Enomoto speaks and writes English and Spanish.	http://oq83.jp/indexEN.php Email: overseas@oq83.jp
	Sayoshi.com (see below) also has an online store serviced by Sankei.	https://www.sayoshi.com/stores/
	At time of writing, Sankei is in the process of opening an Amazon account to sell Ontake and moxa.	Amazon.com
Wakakusa moxa wool	Wakakusa moxa is available in the US, Australia, and Europe but is slightly too good (and too expensive) for the job. Myojo is preferable (see above)	
Chinese green moxa wool	This grade of Chinese moxa is not suitable for Ontake.	

METRONOMES

There are many metronome apps on the market. What is most important is the ability to save playlists, so that you can jump effortlessly from one frequency to another, and a selection of natural sounds. No free app has these features, so you should invest in one of the paid versions. All these three are available in Google Play and the App Store.

Tempo Pro, by Frozen Ape	Reliable, paid version with different sound sets and playlists. The IOS version has a built-in volume slider, but the Google App does not.
Metronome, by Onyx Apps	Paid upgrades include sound sets and playlist functions.
Metronome +, by Dynamic App Design LLC	Paid version has many bells and whistles, perhaps more than you will need for meridian frequency moxibustion.

JET LIGHTERS

Jet lighters can be found in any smoking, pipe, or tobacco shop, or any "head shop" selling alternative smoking equipment. They are easily found online on Amazon or eBay.

UV CABINETS

General	Available online or in most spa or hair care supply stores.
VRay UV Steriliser https://www.indiegogo.com/products/vray-simple-strong-and-sleek-uvc-sterilizer	This one, recommended by an Ontake student, seems more high-powered and effective than most. If this is unavailable, simply search online for "VRay UV Steriliser". The manufacturer is in Korea.

ONLINE RESOURCES

https://web.facebook.com/groups/ontake/	Facebook group dedicated to Ontake. You can bring your questions and thoughts to the Ontake community here.
www.youtube.com/theontakechannel	Much of the material in this book is demonstrated here, with new material added periodically.
www.sayoshi.com/	An online directory of people practising JAM of all styles, with an online store and options to create events, publish articles, and chat in forums about your style of acupuncture.
www.youtube.com/sayoshitv	Interviews by the author with various experts in JAM.

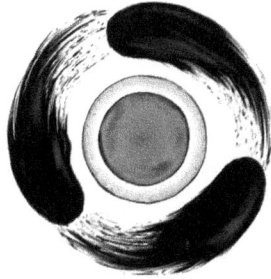

ACKNOWLEDGEMENTS

I must thank Hiroshi Enomoto from Sankei acupuncture suppliers in Tokyo for my introduction to Ontake. It was love at first sight! I use bamboo every day in my clinic and am amazed by its versatility as a therapeutic tool and the rapid changes it can bring about. During my honeymoon period with Ontake in 2010, I developed many of the core techniques of meridian frequency moxibustion, adapting concepts from different Japanese acupuncture styles already shown to be effective.

This resulted in a joyful and ebullient ten-thousand-word paper that I sent to Mr Enomoto, who forwarded it straight to Junji Mizutani at the *North American Journal of Oriental Medicine* (*NAJOM*). I must also thank Mr Mizutani, not just for commissioning a series of articles about Ontake for *NAJOM*, but whose own writings about Press Moxa inspired me.

I would also like to thank my clinical assistant Ryo Izawa, who patiently researched, translated, and summarised huge amounts of source material in Japanese for this book and my next one on Hirata Zones. Ryo also arranged meetings and interviews with practitioners in Japan that would otherwise not have been possible.

No work of mine ever goes far without feedback and guidance from my long-term teaching partner Marian Fixler, who arranged the first workshops in the UK for Ontake, helped me refine and clarify its key teaching concepts and suggested the title of this book. The same goes for my other partners in moxibustion crime, Felip Caudet and Reza Gunawan, whose passion for acupuncture and moxibustion led to many helpful edits to this manuscript.

Warmest thanks are due to my teacher Junko Ida—whose moxa technique inspired me and who, together with Stephen Birch, introduced me not just to the work of Dr Manaka but to the Toyohari Association of Japan and the subtleties of meridian therapy and its blind instructors. All the theories and innovations that I have presented in this book rest on the shoulders of giants.

A final thank you is due to the online community at Self-Publishing School, who helped me edit, produce, and launch this book.

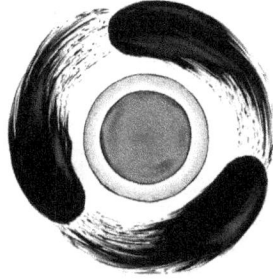

ABOUT THE AUTHOR

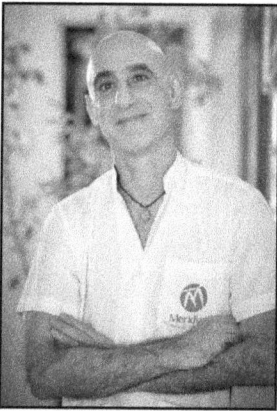

British acupuncturist Oran Kivity trained in Europe, China, and Japan. He ran a busy London practice from 1987 to 2004, and in 2000, he was a founder member of Toyohari UK, the British branch of the Toyohari Association of Japan.

He lectured in acupuncture at the University of Westminster in London from 1994 to 2004 and was a teaching assistant for Stephen Birch, one of the foremost authorities on acupuncture, both in Europe and in South East Asia. Oran's workshops are lively and informative, with a focus on hands-on practice.

Oran moved to Malaysia in 2005 where he practises, writes, teaches, and is the founder of Sayoshi.com, the online directory for all styles of Japanese acupuncture.

Send a Signal?

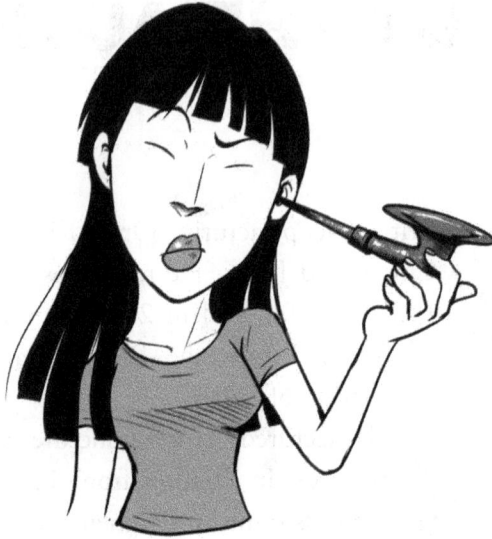

Thank You for Reading My Book!

I really appreciate feedback, and I'd love to hear what you have to say.

To make the next version of this book and my future books better, I need your input.

Please leave me an honest review on Amazon, letting me know what you thought of the content, the writing, and the illustrations.

Thanks so much!

Oran Kivity

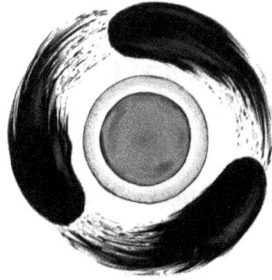

BIBLIOGRAPHY

Auteroche, B. (1992). *Acupuncture and Moxibustion: A Guide to Clinical Practice*. Edinburgh: Churchill Livingstone.

Baek, S. (1990). *Classical Moxibustion Skills in Contemporary Clinical Practice*. Boulder, CO: Blue Poppy Press.

Bensky D., O'Connor, J, (1996). *Acupuncture–A Comprehensive Text*, Shanghai, College of Traditional Medicine Hardcover

Birch, S. (2009). Dr Manaka Yoshio's Insights and Contributions to the Field of TEAM. *NAJOM Special Issue: In Memory of Dr Manaka Yoshio, 16*(47), p.18.

Birch, S. (2018, May 30). Interview by Oran Kivity with Stephen Birch, Junji Mizutani, and Brenda Loew. Retrieved from https://youtu.be/aoN3bwXmacY

Birch, S. (2016). *Shonishin Japanese Pediatric Acupuncture*. Stuttgart: Thieme.

Birch, S., & Felt, R. (1999). *Understanding Acupuncture*. Edinburgh: Churchill Livingstone.

Birch, S., & Ida, J. (1998) *Japanese Acupuncture: A Clinical Guide*. Brookline: Paradigm Publications.

Chant, B., Madison, J., Coop, P., & Dieberg, G. (2017). Beliefs and values in Japanese acupuncture: an ethnography of Japanese trained acupuncture practitioners in Japan. *Integrative Medicine Research, 6*(3), 260–268. http://doi.org/10.1016/j.imr.2017.07.001

Chen, C. (1975). *Essence of Acupuncture Therapy as Based on Yi King and Computers*. Taiwan: International Acupuncture Congress.

Dale, R. (1999). The Systems, Holograms and Theory of Micro-Acupuncture *American Journal of Acupuncture, 27*(3-4), 207–42.

Dann, J. (2009). Editorial. *NAJOM, 16*(47).

Deadman, P., Al-Khafaji, M., & Baker, K., (1998). *A Manual of Acupuncture*. East Sussex, England: Journal of Chinese Medicine Publications,

Enomoto, H. (2010, April 13). (Personal correspondence).

Flaws, B., (1983). *The Path of Pregnancy: Classical Chinese Medical Perspectives on Conception, Pregnancy, Delivery, and Postpartum Care.* Brookline: Paradigm Publications.

Fukushima, K. (1991). *Meridian Therapy.* Tokyo: Toyo Hari Medical Association.

Fukushima, T. (2011) *Johaibu Tokumyaku Goketsu.* Retrieved from http://www. human-world.co.jp/ahaki_world/newsitem/11/0427/110427_2_kanwa.html

Hashimoto, K., & Kawakami, Y. (1983). *Sotai: Balance and Health Through Natural Movement.* Tokyo: Japan Publications Inc.

Hecker, H., Steveling, A., & Peuker, E. (2005). *Microsystems Acupuncture: The Complete Guide: Ear-Scalp-Mouth-Hand.* Stuttgart: Thieme,

Honda, S. (2017). Ontake and Iron Stick Moxibustion. *NAJOM, 24*(69).

Hirata-shiki Nesshin Ryoho Setsumeisho (Hirata-style Warm Needle Therapy Instruction Booklet. Tokyo: Kokusai Nihon Onnetsu Ryoho Kenkyukai (International Japanese Thermotherapy).

Ikeda, M., *Zukai Shinkyu Igaku Nyumon,* quoted in Shudo, D. (1990). *Japanese Classical Acupuncture: Introduction to Meridian Therapy.* Seattle: Eastland Press.

Kivity, O., (2018). Japanese Acupuncture and Moxibustion—What's So Unique? *European Journal of Oriental Medicine, 9*(2).

Kivity, O. (Ed.). (2007). Kikei Nuggets, *Keiraku Chiryo – International Toyohari News,* p.39.

Maciocia, G. (1989). *The Foundations of Chinese Medicine: A Comprehensive Text for Acupuncturists and Herbalists.* Edinburgh: Churchill Livingstone.

Maciocia, G. (1994). *The Practice of Chinese Medicine: The Treatment of Diseases with Acupuncture and Chinese Herbs.* Edinburgh: Churchill Livingstone.

Manaka, Y., (2009). The Concept of Meridians from a Systems Perspective. *NAJOM Special Issue: In Memory of Dr Manaka Yoshio, 16*(47), p. 28.

Manaka, Y., Itaya, K., & Birch, S. (1995). *Chasing the Dragon's Tail: The Theory and Practice of Acupuncture in the Work of Yoshio Manaka.* Brookline: Paradigm Publications.

Manaka, Y., & Urquhart, I., (1972). *The Layman's Guide to Acupuncture.* New York: Weatherhill.

Matsumoto, K., & Birch, S. (1986). *Extraordinary Vessels.* Brookline: Paradigm Publications.

Matsumoto, K., & Birch, S. (1988). *Hara Diagnosis: Reflections on the Sea.* Brookline: Paradigm Publications.

Matsunaga, S., & Ohashi, W. (2001). *Zen Shiatsu: How to Harmonize Yin and Yang for Better Health.* Tokyo: Japan Publications.

McCann, H. (2014). *Pricking the Vessels: Bloodletting Therapy in Chinese Medicine.* London: Singing Dragon.

McCann, H., & Ross, H., (2015). *Practical Atlas of Tung's Acupuncture*. Germany: Verlag Muller & Steinicke.

Mizutani, J. (2018, May 30). Interview by Oran Kivity with Stephen Birch, Junji Mizutani, and Brenda Loew. Retrieved from https://youtu.be/aoN3bwXmacY

Mizutani, J. (1998). Practical Moxibustion Therapy. *North American Journal of Oriental Medicine*. Canada.

Movsessian, P. (2017). Sensitive Patients. *Keiraku Chiryo – International Toyohari News, 11*, p. 8.

Nakayama, T. (2017). Hiesho-Oversensitivity to the Cold. *Keiraku Chiryo – International Toyohari News*.

Ni, M. (1995). *The Yellow Emperors Classic of Medicine: A New Translation of the Neijing Suwen with Commentary*. Boston, MA: Shambhala.

Rosales-Alexander, J., Aznar, J. B., & Magro-Checa, C. (2014). Calcium Pyrophosphate Crystal Deposition Disease: Diagnosis and Treatment. *Open Access Rheumatology: Research and Reviews, 39*. DOI:10.2147/oarrr.s39039

Shinma H., (2012). *Take Zutsu Onkyu, (Bamboo Tube Moxibustion)*. Tokyo: Kyuho Rinsho Kenkyukai.

Shinma, H. (2016). *The Treasure Book of Points Fukaya Kyu*. Tokyo: Hideo Shinma.

Shudo, D. (1990). *Japanese Classical Acupuncture: Introduction to Meridian Therapy*. Seattle: Eastland Press.

Tan, R. T. (2007). *Acupuncture 1, 2, 3*. San Diego, CA: R. Tan.

Tsuboi, K., (2008). The Application of Sanshin Technique According to The Determination of Kyojitsu, *Keiraku Chiryo – International Toyohari News*.

Wang, J.Y., & Robertson, J.D. (2008). *Applied Channel Theory in Chinese Medicine*. Seattle: Eastland Press, Inc.

Yamashita, M. (1992). *Shinkyuchiryogaku (Acupuncture and Moxibustion Therapy)*, Tokyo, Ishiyaku Shuppan.

Young, M. (2012). *The Moon over Matsushima: Insights into Moxa and Mugwort*. United Kingdom: Godiva Books.

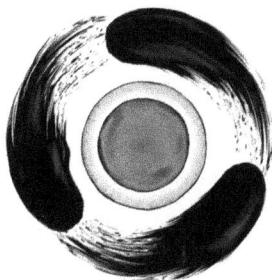

Index

www.ingramcontent.com/pod-product-compliance
Lightning Source LLC
Chambersburg PA
CBHW080619030426
42336CB00018B/3020

9 781916 327900